Joey Green's

Supermarket Spa

Also by Joey Green

Joey Green's

Supermarket Spa

Hundreds of Easy Ways
to Pamper Yourself
Using Brand-Name Products
You've Already Got Around the House

Joey Green

Copyright © 2005 by Joey Green

First published in the USA in 2005 by
Fair Winds Press, a member of Quayside Publishing Group
33 Commercial Street
Gloucester, MA 01930

09 08 07 06 05   1 2 3 4 5

ISBN 1-59233-171-8

Library of Congress Cataloging-in-Publication Data available

Cover design by Laura McFadden
Book design by Joey Green
Photography by Joey Green

Printed and bound in Canada

For my two beautiful daughters,
Ashley and Julia

Ingredients

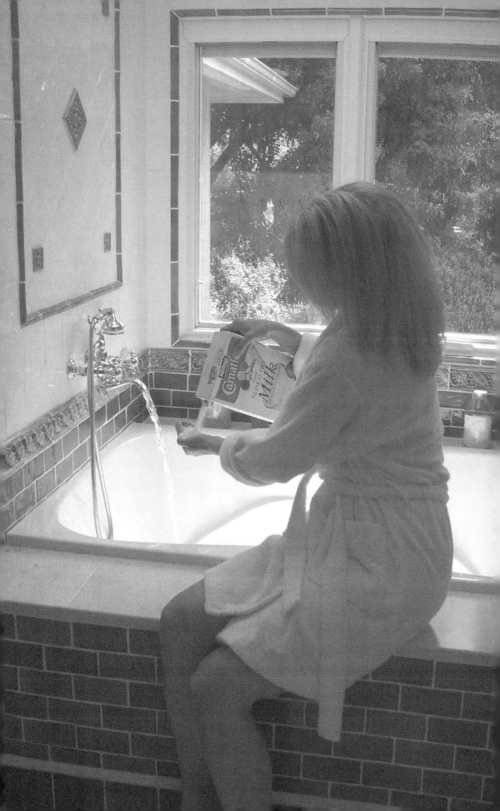

But First a Word from our Sponsor

Step into any "bath and body" boutique at your local shopping mall, pick up a jar of bath salts, a bottle of shampoo, or a tube of hand cream, and look at the price tag. You'll quickly discover that nearly every item in the store sells for an average price of fifteen dollars.

At my local "bath and body" boutique, I was amazed to learn that an eight-ounce jar of milk-bath powder (a fancy name for powdered milk) costs sixteen dollars. Meanwhile, at the grocery store, a box of Carnation NonFat Dry Milk costs less than ten dollars and contains more than three times as much powdered milk.

Why does the small jar at the boutique cost so much more? After all, powdered milk is powdered milk. What you're really paying for at the boutique is the decorative jar, the pretentious label, and the store's comforting ambience, perfumed aromas, and piped-in new-age music. You're being suckered into buying powdered milk for five times the supermarket price.

Skin-care companies aggressively market products "guaranteed" to soften and tighten skin, eliminate wrinkles, and make you feel younger—just because they contain some unique ingredient or secret formula. Most of their claims are impossible to verify, and the "secret formulas" are actually based on age-old recipes that go all the way back to ancient Egypt and Greece.

The truth is: You don't have to spend a fortune to pamper yourself with skin-care products or enjoy a luxurious spa treatment. Using common brand-name products purchased at the supermarket, you can duplicate the posh products sold at "bath and body" boutiques—mud packs, brown sugar exfoliants, sea salt—for just pennies. And you can easily pamper yourself at home with lavish spa treatments—facials, steam baths, manicures, body wraps—to make yourself feel and look cleansed and renewed.

Eighteen years ago, while backpacking around the world on a shoestring budget, I immersed myself at the world-renowned spa in Baden-Baden, Germany; experienced traditional Thai massage in Chiang Mai, Thailand; soaked in therapeutic hot springs at Termas de Palguín, Chilé; and witnessed mud therapy at a spa on the Dead Sea in Israel. Ever since then, I've yearned to unlock the secret formulas for all those rubs, scrubs, cleansers, and toners. I grew determined to find inexpensive and simple ways to make invigorating massage oils, sumptuous aromatherapy treatments, and soothing bath salts—using ordinary household products—so I could revitalize my entire being in the comfort of my own home.

And so, I visited bath and body stores in Beverly Hills, journeyed to exclusive spas in Palm Springs and Murietta Hot Springs, and experimented with scores of brand-name products we all know and love. I coated my body with French's Mustard, wrapped myself in Saran Wrap, conditioned my hair with Cheez Whiz, and gave myself a facial with Phillips' Milk of Magnesia. And then (after showering, of course), I locked myself in the library to unearth a treasure trove of unique beauty secrets for do-it-yourself moisturizers, lotions, liniments, and shampoos—using brand-name products you probably already have in your kitchen.

But I had to know more. What exactly is witch hazel? Is Tiger Balm made from tigers? Who was the actress who played Madge the Manicurist, and what possessed her to soak her customers' fingernails in Palmolive? Who is Betty Crocker? And just how did BenGay get its name?

This book is the result of my obsessive quest into the world of self-indulgence. Inside you'll discover a plethora of practical yet unusual ways to restore, enrich, immerse, and recharge yourself—along with plenty of fun facts—so you, too, will have all the tools you need to reenergize your body, mind, and soul. Pardon me now while I go detoxify.

Aromatherapy

■ **BenGay.** Rub some BenGay on the back of your neck or place a dollop on a cotton ball and set on a saucer as aromatherapy. The menthol in BenGay provides an invigorating scent.

■ **Bounce.** Tape a sheet of Bounce Classic to the front of a fan or over an air-conditioning vent and turn it on to fill the area with the soothing scent of oleander. You can also place a Bounce dryer sheet in the sun visor of your car or under the seat, in a wastebasket, in a drawer, or behind books on a shelf.

■ **Crayola Crayons.** Keep a box of Crayola Crayons on hand and whenever you feel down-and-out, anxious, or tense, simply open the box and smell the crayons. The scent of Crayola Crayons is among the twenty most recognizable to American adults, and the nostalgic aroma instantly triggers a calming sense of peace and security, reminiscent of all the joys of childhood.

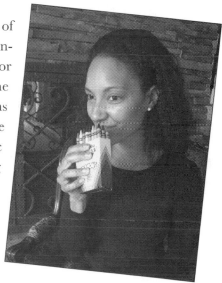

■ **Dr. Bronner's Peppermint Soap.** Add a few drops of Dr. Bronner's Peppermint Soap to your bathwater as aromatherapy to energize your being.

■ **Ivory Soap.** Unwrap a bar of Ivory Soap and place it on a desk, table, or countertop to freshen the air with the calming nostalgic scent of coconut oil, palm oil, and a light fragrance, catapulting your memory back to the innocence of childhood, when you played in the bath with a floating bar of soap.

■ **Johnson's Baby Oil.** For an aromatic bath, mix one-quarter cup Johnson's Baby Oil with a few drops of your favorite perfume or cologne and pour the mixture into your bathwater.

■ **L'eggs Sheer Energy Panty Hose.** Cut off the foot from a clean, used pair of L'eggs Panty Hose, fill with rose petals from your flower bed, and tie a knot in the nylon. Set the sachet on a tabletop, place it in a drawer, or hang it from a lamp.

■ **McCormick Basil Leaves** and **L'eggs Sheer Energy Panty Hose.** Cut off the foot from a clean, used pair of L'eggs Panty Hose, fill with McCormick Basil Leaves, and tie a knot in the nylon. Tie the basil sachet to the spigot, letting it dangle in the flow of water as the tub fills with warm water. Or drop the sachet into the bathwater to brew like a tea bag. Give yourself a long soak in the bathtub, letting the invigorating aroma of basil uplift your soul and improve your concentration. (Do not soak in a basil bath if you are pregnant.)

■ **McCormick Pure Lemon Extract.** Adding a few drops of McCormick Pure Lemon Extract to your bathwater will help clarify your emotions, refresh your spirits, and invigorate your soul. Or saturate a cotton ball with lemon extract (or place a few drops on a tissue) and set on a saucer as aromatherapy to rejuvenate you.

■ **McCormick Pure Orange Extract.** Add a few drops of McCormick Pure Orange Extract to your bathwater and enjoy a long soak to relief stress and revive your spirits. Or saturate a cotton ball with orange extract (or place a few drops on a tissue) and set on a saucer as aromatherapy to lift your spirits.

■ **McCormick Pure Peppermint Extract.** Energize your being and clarify your mind by adding a few drops of McCormick Pure Peppermint Extract to your bathwater. Or saturate a cotton ball with peppermint (or place a few drops on a tissue) and set on a saucer as aromatherapy to calm your nerves and help bring relief from a headache.

■ **McCormiok Pure Vanilla Extract.** Soak a cotton ball in vanilla extract (or place a few drops on a tissue) and set on a saucer as aromatherapy to soothe your nerves. Or place a drop of vanilla extract on your hairbrush.

■ **Mennen Speed Stick.** Apply Mennen Speed Stick to an incandescent light bulb and then turn on the lamp. The heat from the light bulb will slowly melt the deodorant, filling the air in the room with the uplifting scent of, well, deodorant. Or simply remove the cap and place a Speed Stick on a desk or under the seat of your car. Or cut off a chunk and place it on a saucer.

■ **Noxzema.** Rub a dab of Noxzema on your chest to allow the camphor, menthol, and eucalyptus oil to provide soothing and calming aromatherapy.

■ **ReaLemon.** Saturate a cotton ball with ReaLemon lemon juice (or place a few drops on a tissue) and set on a saucer as aromatherapy to brighten your state of mind.

■ **Tiger Balm.** Rub a dab of Tiger Balm into your temples or on your forehead between your eyebrows. Tiger Balm contains camphor, menthol, cajeput oil, and clove oil, which calm your nerves while simultaneously perking up your mood.

■ **Vicks VapoRub.** You can rub Vick's VapoRub on your chest and neck, set an open jar on your desk, or place a dollop of the gel in the medicine chamber on a Vicks Vaporizer to add the aroma to the steam. Vicks VapoRub contains the invigorating and energizing aromas of camphor, menthol, and eucalyptus oil.

Immerse Yourself

■ Aromas trigger memories and emotional responses, and certain oils can be used to relieve stress, depression, and fatigue.

■ Many ancient civilizations burned plants and incense during ritual practices to offer the scent to their God or gods.

■ The word aromatherapy means "smell therapy" and was first coined by French chemist René-Maurice Gattefosse, who used the technique to help heal wounded soldiers during World War I.

■ Aromatherapy uses essential oils that capture the scents from flowers, herbs, trees, and other plants for medicinal and therapeutic purposes.

■ The word perfume stems from the Latin word *perfumum*, which means "through smoke," referring to the burning of incense.

■ Scholars believe that tenth century Arab physician Avicenna discovered the process for extracting or distilling essential oils from plants.

■ Inhaling the gaseous molecules of a fragrance triggers the brain to release endorphins and pheromones, stimulating or calming the body.

■ You can absorb aromatherapy oils through the skin (by massage, through creams and lotions, or by adding the oils to your bath) or inhale them through the olfactory system.

■ While essential oils can be purchased through health food stores, drug stores, and mail order catalogs, you can also use several food extracts sold at the grocery store.

■ In the Biblical book of Exodus, God commands Moses to make a holy anointing oil from myrrh, cinnamon, calamus, cassia, and olive oils.

Essential Oils

Purists insist that true aromatherapy requires the use of essential oils. For authentic aromatherapy, simply add essential oils (available at health food stores) to your bath, inhale them, or massage them into your skin. For an aromatherapy bath, dilute five to ten drops of any of the following essential oils (individually or in combination) with two teaspoons sweet almond oil and then add the solution to warm bathwater and swirl it around. You can inhale essential oils by simply placing a few drops on a handkerchief and breathing. Or you can add ten drops into a pan of boiling water, cover your head with a thick towel, and breathe in deeply for about ten minutes (unless you have asthma). Or you can blend a few drops of various essential oils into a carrier oil (such as International Collection Sweet Almond Oil or Grapeola Grape Seed Oil) and massage into the skin. The chart below lists essential oils by their therapeutic affects.

CALMING	UPLIFTING	STIMULATING
Chamomile	Bergamot	Basil*
Frankincense	Clary sage*	Birch
Jasmine	Coriander	Cardamom
Lavender	Cypress	Cinnamon†
Lemon balm△	Geranium	Clove†
Marjoram*	Grapefruit△	Eucalyptus
Neroli	Mandarin△	Ginger
Palmarosa	Orange△	Juniper*
Rose	Tangerine△	Lemon△
Sandalwood	Tea tree*	Mint
Vetiver	Ylang-ylang	Nutmeg
		Peppermint
		Pine
		Rosemary*

*Do not use during pregnancy.
† Do not use on skin.
△ Do not apply citrus oils directly to the skin before going out in the sun, otherwise your skin will be more prone to sunburn.

Baths

■ Arm & Hammer Baking Soda. Give yourself soft, smooth-feeling skin and a relaxing bath by dissolving one-half cup Arm & Hammer Baking Soda in a bathtub filled with warm water.

■ Carnation NonFat Dry Milk. For a luxurious milk bath worthy of Cleopatra, add one handful Carnation NonFat Dry Milk powder to warm running bathwater. The lactic acid in the milk softens the skin, and the proteins leave the skin feeling silky smooth and rejuvenated.

■ Carnation NonFat Dry Milk, Kingsford's Corn Starch, and **McCormick Pure Vanilla Extract.** Mix one-half cup Carnation NonFat Dry Milk, one-quarter cup Kingsford's Corn Starch, and one teaspoon McCormick Pure Vanilla Extract. Pour the mixture into running bathwater and soak for twenty minutes to soften skin and enjoy the soothing aroma of vanilla.

■ Castor Oil. Restore natural oils to dry skin by adding a few drops of castor oil (no more than two teaspoons) to your bathwater, moisturizing your skin.

■ Clairol Herbal Essences Shampoo. Adding a capful of Clairol Herbal Essences Shampoo to running bathwater yields a luxurious, aromatic, relaxing, and 99 percent all-natural bubble bath. The shampoo also prevents a ring around the tub.

■ Coppertone. Add two tablespoons Coppertone to a warm bath as a moisturizing bath oil.

■ **Dynasty Sesame Seed Oil.** Restore natural oils to dry skin by adding a few drops of Dynasty Sesame Seed Oil (no more than two teaspoons) to your bathwater, moisturizing your skin.

■ **Epsom Salt.** Add one cup Epsom Salt to warm bathwater and soak for more than fifteen minutes to soothe tired muscles.

■ **French's Mustard** and **Epsom Salt.** Add six tablespoons French's Mustard and one handful Epsom Salt into running bathwater as it fill the tub. The soothing, rejuvenating mustard bath, combined with the magnesium sulfate of the Epsom Salt, eases kinks and stiffness in your muscles.

■ **Hain Safflower Oil.** If you have oily skin, give yourself a moisturizing bath by adding a few drops of Hain Safflower Oil (no more than two teaspoons) to your bathwater.

■ **Heinz Apple Cider Vinegar.** Adding one cup Heinz Apple Cider Vinegar—which contains iron, phosphorous, potassium, magnesium, and sodium—to bathwater softens skin and helps restore its natural acid balance. Soak for roughly twenty minutes to give the vinegar sufficient time to do its magic.

■ **Huggies Baby Wipes.** If you're unable to shower or bathe, give yourself a sponge bath with Huggies Baby Wipes, cleansing grime from your skin and leaving you feeling refreshed.

■ **International Collection Sweet Almond Oil.** Give normal skin a moisturizing bath by adding a few drops of almond oil (no more than two teaspoons) to your bathwater.

■ **Ivory Dishwashing Liquid, Wesson Vegetable Oil, McCormick Food Coloring, Morton Rock Salt, Reynolds Cut-Rite Wax Paper, McCormick Pure Almond Extract,** and **Ziploc Storage**

Bags. Make a foaming bath salt by mixing together one-half cup Ivory Dishwashing Liquid, one tablespoon Wesson Vegetable Oil, and a few drops of any color McCormick Food Coloring you desire. Put six cups Morton Rock Salt into a bowl, pour the soapy solution over the salt, and stir well. Spread the coated salt on a cookie sheet covered with Reynolds Cut-Rite Waxed paper. Let dry, sprinkle with two teaspoons McCormick Pure Almond Extract, and store in Ziploc Storage Bags.

■ **Johnson's Baby Oil.** Adding a few drops of Johnson's Baby Oil to your bathwater creates a lavish bath that moisturizes and softens your skin.

■ **L'eggs Sheer Energy Panty Hose.** For a soothing, aromatic bath, cut off one foot from a pair of clean, used L'eggs Sheer Energy Panty Hose, fill the foot with the herb of your choice (lavender, mint, orange peel, lemon rind, rosemary, Quaker Oats, Lipton Chamomile Tea leaves), tie a knot in the open end, and hang it from the faucet in the bathtub under running bathwater.

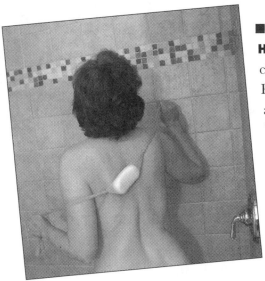

■ **L'eggs Sheer Energy Panty Hose.** Cut off the leg of a pair of clean, used L'eggs Sheer Energy Panty Hose, insert a bar of soap at the knee, tie a knot around both ends of the soap, and use the panty hose to wash your back in the bath.

■ **Lipton Chamomile Tea Bags.** Fill the bath tub with warm water and drop in three Lipton Chamomile Tea Bags to infuse the room with the aroma of chamomile.

■**Maxwell House Coffee.** Get into an empty bathtub and rub warm, freshly-used Maxwell House Coffee grounds all over your body from the neck down. Wait ten minutes, fill the tub with warm water, and soak in this invigorating coffee bath.

■**Minute Maid Orange Juice.** Add one cup Minute Maid Orange Juice to warm bathwater and soak for twenty minutes to rejuvenate dull skin.

■**Ocean Spray Cranberry Juice Cocktail.** Adding one cup Ocean Spray Cranberry Juice Cocktail to your bathwater helps boost circulation.

■**Pampers.** If you are unable to take a bath, saturate a Pampers disposable diaper with water. The super-absorbent polymer flakes in the Pampers hold three hundred times their weight in liquid, enabling you to use the waterlogged diaper for a sponge bath.

■**Quaker Oat Bran Hot Cereal** and **L'eggs Sheer Energy Panty Hose.** Cut off one foot from a pair of clean, used L'eggs Sheer Energy Panty Hose, fill it with Quaker Oat Bran Hot Cereal (uncooked), tie a knot in the open end, and rub the sachet all over your skin while you take a bath. Bran works as moisturizing exfoliant.

■**ReaLemon** and **Johnson's Baby Oil.** Mix one tablespoon ReaLemon lemon juice and one-half cup Johnson's Baby Oil and add the mixture to your bathwater to soften skin and infuse the air with soothing aromatherapy.

■**Skin-So-Soft.** Adding two tablespoons Skin-So-Soft to a warm bath turns this skin moisturizer into a soothing bath oil.

■**Stayfree Maxi Pads.** If you don't have time to take a bath or shower, saturate a Stayfree Maxi Pad with water and use it as a washcloth to give yourself a sponge bath.

■ **SueBee Honey** and **Heinz White Vinegar.** Add one-quarter cup SueBee Honey and one-quarter cup Heinz White Vinegar to your bathwater to leave your skin feeling baby smooth.

■ **Uncle Ben's Instant Brown Rice** and **L'eggs Sheer Energy Panty Hose.** Cut off one foot from a pair of clean, used L'eggs Sheer Energy Panty Hose, fill the foot with Uncle Ben's Instant Brown Rice, tie a knot in the open end, and rub the sachet all over your skin while you take a bath. Brown rice works as moisturizing exfoliant.

■ **Ziploc Freezer Bags.** Make a waterproof pillow for the bathtub by sealing a Ziploc Freezer Bag securely, leaving a half-inch opening at one end of the "zipper." Inflate the bag, quickly seal the remaining half inch, and place the pillow under your head.

■ **Ziploc Storage Bags.** Missing the plug for the drain in the bathtub? Fill a Ziploc Storage Bag with water and, without sealing it, place over the drain hole. The suction from the drain will hold the plastic bag in place, sealing the drain.

Immerse Yourself

■ Adding a few drops of essential oils to your bath can help detoxify, moisturize, and condition your skin. See page 5 for more information on essential oils.

■ Taking a warm bath on a hot summer day lowers your body temperature and opens your pores, making your feel much cooler.

■ Ancient Egyptian Queen Cleopatra, legendary for her incredibly soft skin, purportedly took daily milk baths in camel milk.

■ Soaking in a bathtub for more than ten minutes reduces stress and anxiety, soothes tense muscles, relives menstrual cramps, eases depression, and facilitates sleep.

■ A warm bath can detoxify your system.

■ Enhance a bath by playing relaxing music and lighting the bathing area with scented candles.

■ During the second century B.C.E., the Romans built massive bath houses, offering a range of spa treatments and including gardens, libraries, gymnasiums, exercise rooms, shops, and lecture halls.

■ The Baths of Caracalla, built in Rome in the third century C.E., could accommodate up to 1,600 bathers at a time.

■ The Romans established the city in England now known as Bath to use the warm springs and mineral waters for therapeutic purposes. Baths built by the Romans remain standing to this day. In the eighteenth century, Bath became a resort for English high society.

■ In Japan, people wash before soaking in tubs of hot water, which are used solely for relaxation.

■ Ancient Hebrews apparently began the practice of bathing for religious purposes, washing themselves after contact with the dead. Women immersed themselves in a mikvah (ritual bath) before getting married, married women immersed themselves in water seven days after their menstrual cycles ended, and converts to Judaism are required to immerse themselves in a mikvah.

■ A person entering the Christian religion is baptized by being dipped in water or sprinkled with water.

■ Hindus consider the Ganges River to be sacred and make pilgrimages to its shores to bathe in the water to purify themselves or cure themselves of illnesses.

■ The Puritans, a group of English Protestant who founded the American colonies in New England, forbid bathing, convinced that nudity lead to promiscuity.

■ Benjamin Franklin brought a slipper tub—a bathtub shaped like a slipper to conceal the bather's body—from Europe to the United States.

Cleansing & Toning

■ **Kleenex Tissues.** To determine whether you have oily or dry skin, tear a single-ply strip from a Kleenex Tissue and press it to your face for a few seconds. Remove the strip of tissue and study it. If you see a greasy stain, you have oily skin. If you do not see any stain, you have dry skin.

■ **ReaLemon** and **Star Olive Oil.** To ascertain whether your skin is oily or dry, mix together four teaspoons ReaLemon, one teaspoon Star Olive Oil, four ounces distilled water, and three ice cubes. Let stand at room temperature until the ice cubes melt completely. Cleanse your face with soap and water, pat dry, then apply the solution to your face. Wait three hours. Dampen a cotton ball in the mixture and wipe it across your forehead. Wipe a second dampened cotton ball over your nose. Wipe a third dampened cotton ball over your chin. If all three cotton balls are darkened, you have oily skin. If all three cotton balls are clean, you have dry skin. If the cotton balls are somewhat dirty, you have a combination.

CLEANSERS

■ **Arm & Hammer Baking Soda.** Make a paste from Arm & Hammer Baking Soda and water, smooth over your face, wait ten minutes, and rinse thoroughly with warm water.

■ **Blue Diamond Whole Natural Almonds, SueBee Honey,** and **ReaLemon.** Finely grind three or four Blue Diamond Whole Natural Almonds. Mix together one tablespoon SueBee Honey, one tablespoon ground almonds, and one-half teaspoon ReaLemon lemon juice. Apply to your face, rubbing gently to cleanse the skin. Rinse clean with warm water.

■ **Campbell's Tomato Juice.** Dab Campbell's Tomato Juice on your face, avoiding your eyes, wait ten minutes, then wash clean with warm water. The lactic acid in the tomato juice helps exfoliate the dead skin cells, leaving your face smooth and soft. Tomato juice also contains the antioxidant lycopene.

■ **Dannon Yogurt, Loriva Extra Sunflower Oil,** and **ReaLemon.** Mix one cup Dannon Plain Yogurt, two tablespoons Loriva Extra Sunflower Oil (optional), and three teaspoons ReaLemon lemon juice in a sealed container. Store in the refrigerator. Apply one teaspoon to your face each morning and night, avoiding your eyes, and massage in circles. Wait ten minutes, then wash clean with warm water followed by cool water. This simple concoction simultaneously cleanses, exfoliates, and moisturizes.

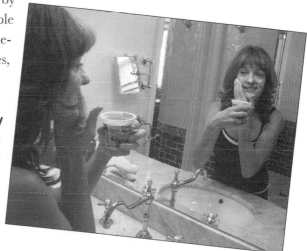

■ **Dannon Blueberry Yogurt.** Mix up the yogurt well and apply the mixture to your face, wait ten minutes, then wash clean with warm water. The lactic acid in the yogurt and the blueberries helps exfoliate the dead skin cells, leaving your face smooth and soft.

■ **Dannon Strawberry Yogurt.** Mix up the yogurt well and apply the mixture to your face, wait ten minutes, then wash clean with warm water. The alpha-hydroxy acid in the strawberries and the lactic acid in the yogurt help exfoliate the dead skin cells, leaving your face smooth and soft.

■ **Dole Pineapple Juice.** Use a cotton ball to apply Dole Pineapple Juice to your face, avoiding your eyes. The various acids in pineapple juice help exfoliate dead skin cells.

■ **Heinz Apple Cider Vinegar.** Use a cotton ball to dab Heinz Apple Cider Vinegar on your face, avoiding your eyes, wait ten minutes, then wash clean with warm water. The malic acid in the vinegar helps exfoliate the dead skin cells, leaving your face smooth and soft.

■ **McCormick Cream of Tartar.** Mix McCormick Cream of Tartar with enough water to make a thick paste. Apply the mixture to your face, wait ten minutes, then wash clean with warm water. The tartaric acid in the cream of tartar helps exfoliate the dead skin cells, leaving your face smooth and soft.

■ **Ocean Spray Cranberry Juice Cocktail.** Soak gauze pads or a cotton handkerchief in Ocean Spray Cranberry Juice Cocktail and place it over your face, avoiding your eyes. Wait ten minutes, then rinse clean with warm water. Cranberry juice gently exfoliates dead skin and fights acne.

■ **Quaker Oats** and **Dannon Yogurt.** Mix one-half cup Quaker Oats and enough Dannon Plain Yogurt to form a paste. Smooth the mixture over your entire face, avoiding your eyes. Wash clean with warm water.

■ **ReaLemon.** Dab ReaLemon lemon juice on your face, avoiding your eyes, wait ten minutes, then wash clean with warm water. The alpha-hydroxy acid in the lemon juice helps exfoliate the dead skin cells, leaving your face smooth and soft. (Using citric acid on your skin makes you more prone to sunburn, so be sure to use sunscreen afterward.)

■ **20 Mule Team Borax** and **Smirnoff Vodka.** To make an effective astringent for normal skin, dissolve one-quarter teaspoon 20 Mule Team Borax in three tablespoons distilled water. Stir well. Add three tablespoons rose water (available at drug stores) and one tablespoon Smirnoff Vodka. Store in a container with a secure lid to prevent the alcohol from evaporating. Wash your face and then apply this homemade astringent with a cotton ball.

■ **Welch's 100% White Grape Juice.** Dab Welch's 100% White Grape Juice (not purple grape juice, which will dye your skin) on your face, avoiding your eyes, wait ten minutes, then wash clean with warm water. The alpha-hydroxy acid and tartaric acid in the grape juice help exfoliate the dead skin cells, leaving your face smooth and soft.

TONERS

■ **Bigelow Plantation Mint Classic Tea Bags.** Steep two Bigelow Plantation Mint Classic Tea Bags in one cup boiling water and refrigerate. Dab the mint tea on your face with a cotton ball to remove oil and grime.

■ **Dickinson's Witch Hazel** and **Mr. Coffee Filters.** For dry to normal skin, use a cotton ball to dab Dickinson's Witch Hazel, straight from the bottle, on your face and let dry. Or mix three-and-a-half cups Dickson's Witch Hazel, one-half cup dried rose petals (from your garden), and five sprigs fresh rosemary. Blend well, store in an airtight container in a dark place for one week. Strain through a Mr. Coffee Filter and store in a sterilized glass bottle, tightly capped. Splash on your face or dab it on with a cotton ball after cleansing skin. Witch hazel, a natural extract from the witch hazel plant, gently cleanses pores deeply.

■ **Dickinson's Witch Hazel** and **ReaLemon.** Mix one-half cup Dickinson's Witch Hazel, one-quarter cup ReaLemon lemon juice, and five drops essential oil of mint and store in a sterilized glass bottle, tightly capped. Using a cotton ball, apply this astringent to oily skin on your face and neck.

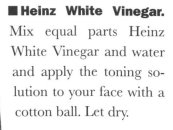

■ **Heinz White Vinegar.** Mix equal parts Heinz White Vinegar and water and apply the toning solution to your face with a cotton ball. Let dry.

■ **Hydrogen Peroxide.** For oily skin, mix hydrogen peroxide with a little water and dab on your skin with a cotton ball.

■ **McCormick Mint Extract** and **McCormick Alum.** For dry skin, mix two drops of McCormick Mint Extract and one-half teaspoon McCormick Alum in one cup distilled water. Apply to your face with a cotton ball and let dry.

■ **Mott's Apple Juice** and **SueBee Honey.** Mix one teaspoon Mott's Apple Juice and one tablespoon SueBee Honey, apply to your face, and wait fifteen minutes. Rinse clean with cool water.

■ **Ocean Spray Cranberry Juice Cocktail, Dickinson's Witch Hazel,** and **Smirnoff Vodka.** Mix two fluid ounces Ocean Spray

Cranberry Juice Cocktail, one tablespoon Dickenson's Witch Hazel, and one tablespoon Smirnoff Vodka. Use a cotton ball to apply to your skin.

■ **ReaLemon.** Lemon juice, a natural astringent, removes any residue and refreshes your face. Add one teaspoon ReaLemon lemon juice to one cup cold water, saturate a cotton ball with the solution, and apply to your face. Let dry and do not rinse. Lemon juice shrinks the pores.

■ **ReaLime.** In a blender, mix one peeled kiwi and two teaspoons ReaLime lime juice. Add an equal amount of water and blend until smooth. Apply to your face with a cotton ball. Refrigerate leftover toner in an airtight container.

■ **Smirnoff Vodka.** For oily skin, clean and tighten your pores by applying Smirnoff Vodka to your face with a cotton ball.

Immerse Yourself

■ Washing your skin helps remove dead cells and stimulates the development of new ones, making your skin look fresh and smooth. If you're under thirty, your skin cells renew themselves quickly. Unfortunately, the older you get, the longer the skin cells take to regenerate, and the resulting buildup of oil and dirt can make skin appear dull and flaky.

■ A simple bar of soap with a pH value between 11 and 14 can be used to cleanse skin. If you have oily skin, use a non-greasy, milky skin cleanser that does not leave a sticky film on the skin. If you have dry skin, use a super fatty cleansing soap with moisture added. If you have sensitive skin, use a fragrance-free mild soap without any unnecessary ingredients.

■ Drinking six to eight glasses of water a day helps replace fluids

DICKINSON'S WITCH HAZEL

Native Americans extracted and distilled compounds from the bark and twigs of witch hazel—a flowering shrub indigenous to the northeastern and central United States—to create an all-natural liquid astringent for use in cleansing, soothing, and healing skin irritations. Native Americans used the witch hazel potion to topically treat minor wounds, abrasions, and other skin ailments, and they drank witch hazel tea to soothe sore muscles and cure lung ailments and diarrhea.

The Native Americans passed on their knowledge of the natural healing powers of witch hazel to early European settlers, who refined the process for extracting essential oils from the pulp material through a distillation process. The name witch hazel refers to the forked twigs of the plant, which at one time were used to locate underground water, in a process commonly known as "water witching."

In 1866, T.N. Dickinson began production of witch hazel extract in Essex, Connecticut, using a formula he obtained from Native Americans. Today, Dickinson Brands is the world's leading marketer and distributor of witch hazel-based products.

in your body, flushes toxins from your system, and enhances your skin—for free.

■ Cleansing removes dirt, sebum, sweat, dead epidermal cells, bacteria, and cosmetics from the skin.

■ After cleansing the skin, rinsing with warm water opens the pores, and rinsing with cool water closes the pores.

■ Toning, an optional step between cleansing and moisturizing, removes any trace of grease or dirt and helps restore the skin's normal pH.

Conditioners & Rinses

■ **Aunt Jemima Original Syrup.** Condition dry hair by massaging Aunt Jemima Original Syrup into your hair and directly into split ends. Cover your hair with a shower cap (or wrap your hair in Saran Wrap) for thirty minutes, then shampoo and rinse well.

■ **Bacardi Rum.** Beat two egg yolks, add one tablespoon Bacardi Rum, and whisk well. Apply to hair, wait thirty minutes, shampoo, and rinse clean.

■ **Budweiser.** To give your hair body, after shampooing, rinse dry hair with Budweiser, wait five minutes, and then rinse clean.

■ **Carnation Evaporated Milk, Heinz White Vinegar,** and **Sue-Bee Honey.** Pour one fourteen-ounce can of Carnation Evaporated Milk into a bowl and add one teaspoon Heinz White Vinegar and one teaspoon SueBee Honey. Mix well, then apply the mixture to dry hair. Wait five minutes, then rinse thoroughly.

■ **Castor Oil.** Treat split ends by rubbing castor oil between your palms and then rubbing your palms over the ends of your hair.

■ **Cheez Whiz.** To condition hair and prevent split ends and frizzies, massage Cheez Whiz into dry hair, cover with a shower cap for thirty minutes, then shampoo and rinse thoroughly.

■ **Coca-Cola.** Give your hair a great shine with the Real Thing. Simply pour a can of Coca-Cola into your hair, work it in well, and then rinse clean with water.

■ **Cool Whip.** Apply Cool Whip to dry hair, wait thirty minutes, rinse clean, and shampoo. The coconut and palm kernel oils in the dessert topping condition hair, giving you a luxurious shine.

■ **Coppertone.** Apply a dollop of Coppertone sunscreen to your hair as a conditioner, then rinse clean. The emollients in Coppertone condition hair.

■ **Dannon Yogurt.** In a bowl, mix five tablespoons Dannon Plain Yogurt and one egg yolk with a whisk to create a creamy paste. Set aside while you shampoo your hair and dry with a towel. Massage the conditioning mixture into your hair, cover with a plastic shower cap (or wrap hair in Saran Wrap), wrap in a warm towel, and wait fifteen minutes. Rinse your hair clean with warm water, followed by a final rinse of cold water. The lecithin in egg yolk helps enrich dry hair, adding volume and body.

■ **Downy Fabric Softener.** If you run out of crème rinse, use a drop of Downy Fabric Softener in your final rinse to leave your hair tangle-free, soft, and smelling April fresh.

■ **Epsom Salt.** Mix three tablespoons of your regular conditioner with three tablespoons Epsom Salt and heat the mixture in a microwave oven. Let cool to the touch, work the warm mixture through your hair, and let set for twenty minutes. Rinse with warm water. The magnesium sulfate helps revitalize dry hair.

■ **Gerber Pears** and **Knox Gelatin.** Mix the contents of one six-ounce jar Gerber Pears and one teaspoon Knox Gelatin powder. After shampooing and rinsing your hair, apply the mixture to your hair and massage into the scalp. Wait fifteen minutes and then shampoo and rinse clean. The pears add texture and volume to hair.

■ **Guinness Extra Stout** and **Star Olive Oil.** Mix one cup Guinness dark beer and one teaspoon Star Olive Oil in a bowl with a whisk. Pour the mixture through your clean hair, massage into the scalp for five minutes, then rinse clean. The beer adds body and volume to your hair, and the olive oil softens and conditions the hair.

■ **Hain Safflower Oil** and **Saran Wrap.** Saturate dry hair with Hain Safflower Oil, cover with Saran Wrap (or a shower cap), wrap in a warm towel, wait two hours, and rinse clean.

■ **Heinz Apple Cider Vinegar.** Mix one cup Heinz Apple Cider Vinegar and two cups water in a sixteen-ounce trigger spray bottle. After shampooing, spray your hair with the mixture. Vinegar adds highlights to brown hair, restores the acid mantle, fights dandruff, and removes soap film and sebum oil—leaving hair looking glossy and feeling smooth.

■ **Heinz White Vinegar.** Rinse oily hair with equal parts Heinz White Vinegar and water.

■ **Heinz White Vinegar.** Make your own scented hair rinse by adding herbs and spices to a bottle of Heinz White Vinegar and letting it stand for two weeks to infuse. Strain the solution through a Mr. Coffee Filter, dilute with equal parts water, and store in a plastic bottle or container. Apply to hair and rinse clean with warm water.

■ **International Collection Sweet Almond Oil.** Put a few drops of International Collection Sweet Almond Oil on your fingertips and rub the oil into your hair. Wait twenty minutes, then shampoo and condition.

■ **Kraft Mayo.** Massage Kraft Mayo into dry hair, let sit for thirty minutes, then rinse several times before shampooing thoroughly. The oil and eggs in the mayonnaise revitalize dry hair and give it a great shine.

■ **Kraft Mayo, Heinz Apple Cider Vinegar,** and **ReaLemon.** Mix one tablespoon Kraft Mayo, two tablespoons Heinz Apple Cider Vinegar, and two tablespoons ReaLemon lemon juice. Work into dry hair, wait twenty minutes, then rinse clean with warm water.

■ **Land O Lakes Butter.** Massage Land O Lakes Butter into dry hair, cover hair with a shower cap (or wrap hair in Saran Wrap) for thirty minutes, then shampoo and rinse thoroughly. Conditioning your hair with butter leaves hair silky soft.

■ **Lipton Tea Bags** and **McCormick Rosemary Leaves.** Brew one cup regular Lipton Tea, add one tablespoon McCormick Rosemary Leaves, and steep for ten minutes. Let cool, pour through your hair, and massage. Rinse clean.

■ **Miracle Whip.** Apply Miracle Whip to dry hair, wait thirty minutes, then rinse several times before shampooing thoroughly. The oils in this miracle treatment revitalize dry hair and give it a great shine.

■ **Nestea.** Mix one quart Nestea according the directions on the jar (using warm water and without adding sugar). Use the tea as a final rinse after shampooing your hair. Nestea gives a natural shine to hair.

■ **Ocean Spray Cranberry Juice Cocktail.** If you're a redhead or brunette, rinsing your hair with one cup Ocean Spray Cranberry Juice Cocktail gives hair a beautiful shine. Rinse clean with one cup cool water.

■ **Pam Cooking Spray.** While standing in a shower stall, lightly spray your hair with Pam Cooking Spray and then run your fingers through your hair. The cooking oil conditions your hair and scalp and gives your hair a wonderful shine.

■ **ReaLemon.** For oily hair, mix equal parts ReaLemon lemon juice and water and, after using your regular shampoo, rinse your hair with the lemon solution.

■ **Reddi-wip.** If you run out of crème rinse, use Reddi-wip whipped cream. Fill the cupped palm of your hand with Reddi-wip, apply to your hair, cover with a shower cap (or wrap your hair in Saran Wrap), wait fifteen minutes, then rinse well and shampoo.

■ **Silk Soy Milk** and **Kingsford's Corn Starch.** Mix one-half cup Silk Soy Milk and three tablespoons Kingsford's Corn Starch and comb the mixture through wet hair. Wait ten minutes and then rinse clean. The soy milk nourishes the cuticle, rejuvenating brittle hair.

■ **Smirnoff Vodka** and **Canada Dry Club Soda.** Mix two tablespoons Smirnoff Vodka and one cup Canada Dry Club Soda. Use as a final rinse to wash away residue from shampoo and other hair products.

■ **Smirnoff Vodka** and **ReaLemon.** Mix one-quarter cup Smirnoff Vodka, two teaspoons ReaLemon lemon juice, and one cup distilled water. Before shampooing, pour this mixture through your hair to remove styling-product buildup.

■ **Star Olive Oil.** Pour a few drops of Star Olive Oil in the cupped palm your hand, rub your hands together, and then run your hands through your hair. The olive oil conditions your hair and scalp and gives your hair a wonderful shine.

■ **Star Olive Oil.** Warm one-half cup Star Olive Oil in a microwave oven until slightly warm to the touch. Treat dry hair and split ends by massaging the olive oil into your hair and then wrapping it in a towel for five minutes before shampooing and conditioning.

■ **SueBee Honey.** To soften your hair and give it a great shine, mix one-half cup SueBee Honey and one egg. Apply the mixture to dry hair, comb it through, then wait one hour. Rinse clean.

■ **SueBee Honey** and **Star Olive Oil.** Mix one tablespoon SueBee Honey and two teaspoons Star Olive Oil. Warm the mixture in a microwave oven, then use your fingers to rub the sticky concoction through your hair. Soak a towel in hot water, wring out completely, and wrap around your head for twenty minutes. Then shampoo as usual, lathering well to remove the olive oil, leaving your hair with more body and fullness.

■ **SueBee Honey, Bacardi Rum,** and **Heinz Apple Cider Vinegar.** In a microwave oven, warm one-quarter cup SueBee Honey. Let cool to the touch and apply to your roots. Mix one ounce Bacardi Rum and two egg yolks and work into the roots of your hair. Cover your hair with a shower cap (or wrap your hair in Saran Wrap) for twenty minutes, then rinse with a solution of one ounce Heinz Apple Cider Vinegar and seven ounces water.

■ **Wesson Corn Oil.** Heat three teaspoons Wesson Corn Oil in a microwave oven, massage the warm oil into dry hair, cover with a shower cap (or wrap your hair in Saran Wrap) for thirty minutes, then shampoo and rinse thoroughly.

■ **Wesson Canola Oil, Fleishmann's Margarine, SueBee Honey,** and **Aunt Jemima Original Syrup.** To condition damaged hair, mix one tablespoon each of Wesson Canola Oil, Fleishmann's Margarine, SueBee Honey, and Aunt Jemima Original Syrup. Heat briefly in a microwave oven, massage the warm syrupy mixture into your hair, wait fifteen minutes, then shampoo and rinse well.

Immerse Yourself

■ Conditioners improve the hair's natural sheen by helping to smooth the hair cuticle. A conditioner or crème rinse replaces the oils stripped from the hair by shampooing.

■ Commercial conditions contain "cationic surfactants," which temporarily coat dry and damaged hair.

■ During the day, the hair follicles produce enough sebum (natural hair oil) to adequately coat the first three inches of hair closest to the scalp. Using a conditioner or crème rinse on the first three inches of hair can over-condition that area. Instead, apply the conditioner or crème rinse on hair three inches from the scalp to the ends and comb the conditioner through the hair.

■ Many people neglect to rinse all traces of conditioner from their hair. Be sure to rinse several times, otherwise a residue of conditioner leaves hair dull and limp.

■ Use the deep conditioning treatments listed in this chapter no more than once a week, otherwise a protein-based deep conditioner meant to strengthen and add body could cause your hair to become dry and brittle, and an oil-based deep conditioner could turn your hair limp and lifeless.

Depilatories

■ **C&H Cane Granulated Sugar.** Mix four teaspoons C&H Cane Granulated Sugar with four teaspoons water in a saucepan over low heat. Stir until the sugar dissolves completely and the sugary liquid thickens to the consistency of runny honey. Remove from heat, let cool to body temperature (98.6 degrees Fahrenheit), and, using a spatula, apply the sticky sugar paste to any unwanted hair on your face, legs, or bikini area. Press a strip of clean cotton gauze over the mixture and let harden. In one quick motion, rip the cotton gauze from your skin—in the opposite direction of the hair growth. The gauze and sugar solution will rip the hairs from your skin, which may appear slightly red. Rinse the skin with cold water.

■ **C&H Cane Sugar, SueBee Honey, Rea-Lemon,** and **Kingsford's Corn Starch.** Mix one cup C&H Cane Sugar, one-quarter cup SueBee Honey, and two teaspoons ReaLemon lemon juice in a saucepan and warm over a low heat, until the mixture has the consistency of glue. Allow the mixture to cool to the touch. Dust the area of skin you intend to depilate with Kingsford's Corn Starch to draw out the oil. Using a spatula, spread a thin layer of the warm sugar and honey mixture over the skin, cover with a strip of cotton fabric, and firmly rub the strip in the opposite direction of the hair growth. Grab the fabric end and pull it off quickly against the direction of the hair growth.

■ **Carnation NonFat Dry Milk.** After waxing your eyebrows, bikini area, or legs, apply a solution of Carnation NonFat Dry Milk mixed with warm water (make it slightly more liquid than a paste) and dab on affected areas. Let sit for ten minutes, then rinse.

■ **Dannon Yogurt.** After waxing, soothe irritated skin by applying Dannon Plain Yogurt to the reddened area. Wait fifteen minutes and then rinse clean.

■ **Johnson's Baby Powder.** Before waxing, dust your legs lightly with Johnson's Baby Powder to help the wax adhere to the hairs.

■ **Lipton Tea Bags.** If your skin gets irritated from waxing, apply a dampened Lipton Tea Bag to the affected skin. The tannic acid from the tea relieves the redness and burning pain.

■ **Orajel.** To reduce the pain when plucking your eyebrows, dab on some liquid Orajel first to anesthetize your skin.

■ **ReaLemon** and **SueBee Honey.** To bleach facial hair naturally, mix one tablespoon ReaLemon lemon juice with four teaspoons SueBee honey. Smooth on in the direction of the hair growth, wait fifteen minutes, and rinse clean. Repeat twice a week. (Using citric acid on your skin makes you more prone to sunburn, so be sure to use sunscreen afterward.)

■ **ReaLime.** After waxing, soothe the redness by applying ReaLime lime juice to the irritated skin. (Using citric acid on your skin makes you more prone to sunburn, so be sure to use sunscreen afterward.)

■ **Scotch Packaging Tape.** Press a strip of Scotch Packaging Tape over the area you wish to depilate, then quickly rip off the tape, pulling against the direction of the hair growth. The hair adheres to the tape.

Immerse Yourself

■ Depilatories—available as lotions, creams, roll-ons, mousses, and gels—contain a substance high in pH, such as sodium thioglycolate or calcium thioglycolate, which reacts with the protein structure of hair, dissolving it, including below the skin's surface.

■ Waxing pulls hair out by the root with a "wax"—usually beeswax, rosin, or a sugar mixture—that is spread onto skin and then covered with strips of cloth that are quickly pulled off the skin.

■ Tweezing requires pulling out each individual hair by the root—one by one.

■ Electrolysis kills the hair follicle with an electric current.

■ For laser hair removal, a specially formulated liquid is applied to the skin and absorbed into the hair follicle, where it absorbs the heat from a laser scanned across the skin, destroying the unwanted hair follicle.

■ The average human has approximately two million hair follicles. That's 3,000 to 4,000 hair follicles per square inch of skin.

■ People have used depilatories as far back as 4000 to 3000 B.C.E., when women used "rhusma turcorum," a paste made from orpiment (natural arsenic trisulphide), quicklime, and starch.

■ South American natives used secretions from the Coco de Mono tree to remove hair.

■ Ancient Egyptians removed hair by waxing with a mixture of crushed birds' bones, sycamore gum, and cucumber.

Eyes

■ **Aqua Net Hair Spray** and **Oral-B Toothbrush.** Spray a little Aqua Net Hair Spray on a clean, used Oral-B Toothbrush and brush your eyebrows to keep them in place.

■ **Betty Crocker Potato Buds** and **Lipton Chamomile Tea Bags.** To soothe tired eyes, mix Betty Crocker Buds with enough water to make a thick paste, cut open a used Lipton Chamomile Tea Bag and stir in the wet tea leaves (optional). Apply the paste to closed eyes (making sure to remove contact lenses or any eye makeup beforehand), cover with a washcloth, and relax for twenty minutes. Rinse clean.

■ **Birds Eye Baby Peas.** Ice reduces the swelling of puffy eyes, eases the pain, and constricts the blood vessels to prevent discoloration. Use a plastic bag of frozen Birds Eye Baby Peas as an ice pack around your eyes for ten minutes. If the bags of peas feels too cold, place a paper towel between your skin and the bag. The sack of peas conforms to the shape of your face, and you can refreeze the peas for future ice-pack use. Be sure to label the bag for ice-pack use only. If you want to eat the peas, cook them after they thaw the first time, never after refreezing.

■ **Dickinson's Witch Hazel.** To soothe tired eyes and reduce puffy eyes, dampen cotton pads with Dickinson's Witch Hazel, lie down, and place the pads on your closed eyelids.

■ **Fruit of the Earth Aloe Vera Gel** and **Dynasty Sesame Seed Oil.** Mix two tablespoons Fruit of the Earth Aloe Vera Gel and one tablespoon Dynasty Sesame Seed Oil with a whisk. Apply to the area around your eye with the fingertip of your middle finger in a gentle circular motion. The sesame oil reduces puffiness, and the aloe vera moisturizes the skin.

■ **Gerber Bananas.** To reduce circles under your eyes, spread the contents of one six-ounce jar Gerber Bananas over your clean, dry face, wait ten minutes, and then rinse clean with cool water. The bananas leave your skin feeling soft, and the potassium helps eliminate circles under your eyes.

■ **Jell-O** and **Ziploc Freezer Bags.** To eliminate puffy eyes, prepare Jell-O according to the directions on the box and let cool enough to pour into a Ziploc Freezer Bag until three-quarters full. Seal the bag shut securely and freeze, and you have a homemade, flexible ice pack. When the Jell-O melts, simply refreeze. Place around your eyes for ten minutes to reduce the swelling and constrict the blood vessels to prevent discoloration.

■ **Lipton Tea Bags.** Soothe tired eyes by immersing two Lipton Tea Bags in warm water, squeezing out the excess moisture, and placing them over your closed eyes for twenty minutes. The tannin in the tea reduces the puffiness and revitalizes tired eyes. Chamomile tea bags also help relieve tired eyes.

■ **Orajel.** To reduce the pain when plucking your eyebrows, dab on some liquid Orajel first to anesthetize your skin.

■ **Post-it Notes.** To protect your eyes when using hair spray or coloring your hair, apply Post-it Notes over your eyebrows to create protective awnings.

■ **Preparation H.** Reduce puffy bags under your eyes by carefully rubbing Preparation H into the skin around the eyes. The hemorrhoid ointment acts as a vasoconstrictor and relieves swelling. (Just be careful not to get it in your eyes.)

■ **Quaker Oats.** Soothe puffy eyes by mixing up one-half cup Quaker Oats according to the directions on the canister, chill in the refrigerator, then apply to your closed eyes. Wait ten minutes, then wash clean.

■ **Smirnoff Vodka, Ziploc Freezer Bags,** and **McCormick Food Coloring.** To reduce bags under your eyes, pour one-half cup Smirnoff Vodka and one-half cup water into a Ziploc Freezer Bag (add five drops of blue food coloring for easy identification), and freeze. The alcohol doesn't freeze, but the water does—giving you have a slushy, refreezable ice pack that you can apply around your eyes to soothe puffy eyes.

■ **Uncle Ben's Converted Brand Rice.** Fill a clean sock with uncooked Uncle Ben's Converted Brand Rice (not too compactly). Tie a knot in the end of the sock. Heat the sock in the microwave for a few minutes and then place the warm sock over your closed eyes for ten minutes to relieve any soreness. The sock conforms to the shape of your face.

■ **Vaseline Petroleum Jelly.** Rub a dab of Vaseline Petroleum Jelly over your eyebrows to keep them in place.

■ **Vaseline Petroleum Jelly.** A small dab of Vaseline Petroleum Jelly on your eyelids creates a stylish gleam.

BETTY CROCKER

In 1921, customers inundated the Washburn Crosby Company, maker of Gold Medal Flour, with letters responding to an offer for a free flour-sack pincushion and requesting recipes. Sam Gale, head of the company's advertising department, created a fictional spokeswoman, Betty Crocker (named in honor of a retired company director, William G. Crocker), so that correspondence to housewives could go out with a single spokeswoman's signature. An employee named Florence Lindeberg provided Betty's signature. Employees in the Washburn Crosby test kitchens provided recipes. In 1936, fifteen years after Betty Crocker was first created, artist Neysa McMein painted Betty Crocker's first formal portrait. Betty is now in her seventh incarnation.

Over the years, Betty's inspirational tips have featured such witticism as "If you're going to drink the cider, first you have to peel the apple;" "Sometimes the heart sees what is invisible to the eye;" and "Wealth is what you are, not what you have."

Immerse Yourself

■ Fish do not blink because they do not have eyelids.

■ The giant squid has the largest eyes in the entire animal kingdom, up to eighteen inches in diameter, approximately the size of a volleyball.

■ The pupil in a goat's eye is rectangular.

■ Starfish have five eyes, one at the tip of each arm. These eyes sense light—but cannot see images.

■ Pinocchio is Italian for "pine eyes."

■ The ostrich has the largest eye of any bird. Its eye, nearly two inches in diameter, is bigger than its brain.

■ The average human eyebrow has 450 hairs.

Facials

■ **Albers Corn Meal.** Make a paste from Albers Corn Meal and water, apply to your face, massage well, wait ten minutes, then wash clean with warm water. The corn meal cleanses the skin, absorbing grime.

■ **Bayer Aspirin.** Unless you're allergic to aspirin, grind six Bayer Aspirin into a fine powder using a mortar and pestle. Add just enough water to make a thin paste, dampen your face, and gently massage the paste into your skin, avoiding your eyes. The salicylic acid in the aspirin exfoliates dead skin cells. Rinse clean with warm water.

■ **C&H Cane Sugar** and **Johnson's Baby Shampoo.** Make an exfoliating facial wash by mixing one-quarter cup C&H Cane Sugar, one teaspoon Johnson's Baby Shampoo, and one-quarter cup water. Rub the gritty paste over your face and then wash with warm water, followed by cold water.

■ **Campbell's Tomato Soup** and **Gold Medal Flour.** Mix together the contents of one can Campbell's Tomato Soup with enough Gold Medal Flour to make a thick paste. Apply the paste to your face and neck, wait fifteen minutes, and then rinse clean with warm water. The acids from the tomatoes balance the pH level of the skin, exfoliate dead skin, and tighten pores.

■ **Carnation NonFat Dry Milk.** Mix one-quarter cup Carnation NonFat Dry Milk with enough water to make a thick paste. Apply the milky paste to your face, let dry, then wash off. The lactic acids remove grime and exfoliate dead skin, and the proteins in the milk leave the skin feeling silky smooth.

■ **Cheerios, SueBee Honey,** and **ReaLemon.** In a blender, grind one cup Cheerios into a fine powder. In a bowl, mix the powdered Cheerios with enough SueBee Honey and ReaLemon lemon juice to make a thick paste. Apply the mixture to your face, wait ten minutes, then rinse with warm water. The Cheerios oats absorb oils from the skin, the lemon juice disinfects the pores, and the honey moisturizes the skin.

■ **Colgate Toothpaste.** Squeeze a dollop of Colgate Regular Flavor Toothpaste into the cupped palm your hand, add a few drops of water, and rub your hands together to create a lather. Coat your face with the toothpaste lather, then rinse thoroughly. Toothpaste is a mild abrasive that cleanses the skin and leaves your face feeling minty fresh.

■ **Cool Whip.** For an invigorating and moisturizing facial, cover your face with Cool Whip, wait twenty minutes, and then wash clean with warm water followed by cold water. The coconut and palm kernel oils in Cool Whip moisturize and soothe the skin.

■ **Country Time Lemonade.** Mix one tablespoon Country Time Lemonade powdered drink with enough water to make a thick paste. Massage the lemony paste over your face (avoiding your eyes), wait five minutes, then rinse clean. The gritty paste and citric acid help exfoliate dead skin, leaving your face smooth and soft. (Using citric acid on your skin makes you more prone to sunburn, so be sure to use sunscreen afterward.)

■ **Dannon Peach Yogurt.** To soothe and smooth your skin, mix up one cup Dannon Peach Yogurt and massage it over your face, avoiding your eyes. Wait fifteen minutes, then rinse clean with warm water. The acids in the peaches and lactic acid in the yogurt do the trick.

■ **Dannon Yogurt.** To tighten pores and cleanse skin, spread Dannon Plain Yogurt over your face, wait twenty minutes, then rinse clean with lukewarm water.

■ **Dannon Yogurt.** Mix one tablespoon Dannon Plain Yogurt with one thin slice avocado. Massage the creamy mixture into your face, let sit for twenty minutes, and then rinse with warm water.

■ **Dr. Bronner's Peppermint Soap.** Place a hand towel in a sink filled with hot water and add a dash of Dr. Bronner's Peppermint Soap. Wring out the towel, lay it over your face, and massage with your fingertips. The peppermint oil in the soap rejuvenates and invigorates the skin, increasing circulation.

■ **Elmer's Glue-All.** Using your fingertips or a one-inch paintbrush, coat your face with a thin layer of Elmer's Glue-All (avoiding your eyes). Wait for the glue to dry (approximately twenty minutes), then gently peel it off, exfoliating a thin layer of skin and removing blackheads. Elmer's Glue-All is water soluble, so you can wash it off with warm water should it stick your eyebrows.

■ **French's Mustard.** Apply French's Mustard as a face mask, wait ten minutes, and then rinse clean with warm water, followed by cool water. The mustard stimulates and soothes the skin.

■ **Fruit of the Earth Aloe Vera Gel, SueBee Honey,** and **Kingsford's Corn Starch.** Mix equal parts Fruit of the Earth Aloe Vera Gel and SueBee Honey, blend thoroughly, then stir in enough Kingsford's Corn Starch to thicken the mixture to the consistency of a face cream. Spread the paste on your face, let dry completely, and then rub off with a wet washcloth to gently exfoliate the skin.

■ **Gerber Bananas.** If you have dry skin, spread the contents of one six-ounce jar Gerber Bananas over your clean, dry face, wait ten minutes, and then rinse clean with cool water. The bananas leave your skin feeling soft, and the potassium helps eliminate circles under your eyes.

■ **Gerber Bananas, McCormick Pure Almond Extract,** and **Lipton Chamomile Tea Bags.** Mix the contents of one six-ounce jar Gerber Bananas, one egg yolk, and one teaspoon McCormick Pure Almond Extract. Apply to your face and let dry. Meanwhile, use several Lipton Chamomile Tea Bags to brew a strong pot of chamomile tea by letting the tea bags steep for ten minutes. Allow it to cool. Saturate a washcloth with cool chamomile tea to wash your face, moisturizing the skin.

■ **Gerber Carrots** and **SueBee Honey.** For normal or oily skin, mix the contents of one six-ounce jar Gerber Carrots with five tablespoons SueBee Honey. Apply this antioxidant mask to your face, wait fifteen minutes, then rinse clean with water.

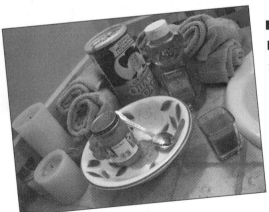

■ **Gerber Peaches, SueBee Honey,** and **Quaker Oats.** For normal skin, mix the contents of one six-ounce jar Gerber Peaches, one tablespoon Sue-Bee Honey, and enough Quaker Oats to create a thick paste. Apply to your face, wait ten minutes, and then rinse well with cool water. Peaches contain large amounts of alpha-hydroxy acids, which gently exfoliate skin, accelerating cell renewal, leading to healthier skin tone. Alpha-hydroxy acids also help soften wrinkles, sun spots, age spots, and blemishes.

■ **Gold Medal Flour, SueBee Honey,** and **Glycerin.** Using a whisk, mix together one-quarter cup Gold Medal Flour, one tablespoon SueBee Honey, one teaspoon glycerin (available at drug stores), and one egg white. Apply the paste to your face and neck, let sit fifteen minutes, and then rinse clean with warm water.

■ **Hennessy Cognac, Carnation NonFat Dry Milk,** and **Rea-Lemon.** Mix one tablespoon Hennessey Cognac, one-quarter cup Carnation NonFat Dry Milk powder, two teaspoons ReaLemon lemon juice, and one whole egg. Apply the mixture to your face, avoiding your eyes, and let dry. Rinse clean with warm water.

■ **Hodgson Mill Oat Bran Flour, C&H Cane Sugar,** and **Dannon Yogurt.** Mix three tablespoons Hodgson Mill Oat Bran Flour, one teaspoon C&H Cane Sugar, and one teaspoon Dannon Plain Yogurt into a paste. Massage this antioxidant solution into your face, wait five minutes, then gently pat dry.

■ **Hunt's Tomato Paste.** Spread Hunt's Tomato Paste over your face, wait ten minutes, then rinse clean and pat dry with a towel. The acids from the tomatoes balance the pH level of the skin, exfoliate dead skin, and tighten pores.

■ **Libby's Pumpkin.** To get your skin silky soft, cover your face with a thin coat of pumpkin, let dry, and then rinse clean. Pumpkin, loaded with vitamin A and fruit acid enzymes, moisturizes and conditions the skin.

■ **Lipton Chamomile Tea Bags, Dynasty Sesame Seed Oil,** and **Wesson Vegetable Oil.** Cut open a Lipton Chamomile Tea Bag and mix the leaves with one tablespoon Dynasty Sesame Seed Oil and one teaspoon Wesson Vegetable Oil. Apply the mixture to your face and neck, remove excess with a tissue, and let set overnight. In the morning, rinse clean with warm water.

■ **Maxwell House Coffee.** Spread warmed, used Maxwell House Coffee ground on your face, wait one minute, then rinse clean with warm water. The caffeine in the coffee tightens the skin.

■ **McCormick Ground Cloves** and **SueBee Honey.** Mix one-quarter teaspoon McCormick Ground Cloves with one-quarter cup SueBee Honey. Apply to your face as a mask, let sit for fifteen minutes, then rinse clean with warm water, followed by cool water.

■ **McCormick Ground Turmeric** and **SueBee Honey.** Mix two tablespoons McCormick Ground Turmeric, two tablespoons warm water, and one tablespoon SueBee Honey. Apply to your face, wait twenty minutes, then rinse clean with warm water.

■ **Minute Maid Orange Juice** and **Dannon Yogurt.** Mix two fluid ounces Minute Maid Orange Juice and one tablespoon Dannon Plain Yogurt and apply the creamy mixture to your face, avoiding your eyes. Wait five minutes. Rinse clean with cool water.

■ **Minute Maid Orange Juice** and **SueBee Honey.** Mix equal parts Minute Maid Orange Juice and SueBee Honey. Apply to your face, avoiding your eyes. Wait five minutes, then rinse clean. The citric acid in the orange juice dries up excess oil, and the honey prevents bacteria from reproducing. (Using citric acid on your skin makes you prone to sunburn, so use sunscreen afterward.)

■ **Miracle Whip.** Give yourself a rejuvenating, moisturizing facial by applying Miracle Whip as a face mask. Leave it on for twenty minutes, then wash off with warm water, followed by cold water. Miracle Whip cleanses the skin and tightens the pores.

■ **Morton Salt.** Fill a trigger-spray bottle with tepid water, add one teaspoon Morton Salt, shake well, and spray the solution on your face. Pat dry with a towel.

■ **Mott's Applesauce.** Rub Mott's Applesauce over your face, wait thirty minutes, and wash with lukewarm water. The applesauce cleans dry skin, and the pectin in the applesauce absorbs excess oil, leaving your skin feeling refreshed.

■ **Mott's Applesauce, Quaker Oats, Albers Corn Meal,** and **SueBee Honey.** Mix four tablespoons Mott's Applesauce, two tablespoons Quaker Oats, one tablespoon Albers Corn Meal, and one tablespoon SueBee Honey into a smooth paste. Apply to your face, avoiding your eyes, massaging in a circular motion. Rinse clean with warm water and pat dry with a towel. The juice in the applesauce tightens pores, the pectin soothes the skin, and the oatmeal and corn meal exfoliate dead skin cells, boosting circulation.

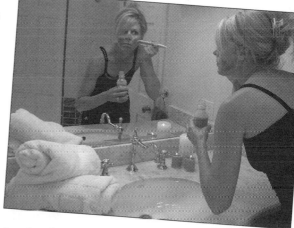

■ **Pepto-Bismol.** Use a cotton ball or a thin gravy brush to cover your face with Pepto-Bismol (avoiding your eyes), let dry, then rinse with cool water to dry the oils from your skin.

■ **Phillips' Milk of Magnesia.** Use a cotton ball to apply Phillips' Milk of Magnesia as a facial mask, let dry for thirty minutes, then rinse off with warm water, followed by cool water. The milk of magnesia absorbs the oils from your skin, while simultaneously cooling the skin, leaving your face minty fresh.

■ **Quaker Oats** and **Albers Corn Meal.** Mix equal parts Quaker Oats and Albers Corn Meal with hot water to make a paste. Let cool to a warm temperature and apply the mixture to your face. Wait ten minutes and then rinse clean with warm water.

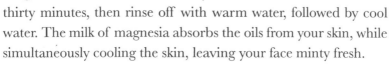

■ **Quaker Oats, Gerber Bananas,** and **SueBee Honey.** For dry skin, cook up one-half cup Quaker Oats (with water) according to the directions on the canister. When the oatmeal cools to the touch, mix with the contents of one six-ounce jar Gerber Bananas, one teaspoon SueBee Honey, and one egg yolk. Apply to your face, wait fifteen minutes, then rinse clean with cool water.

■ **Quaker Oats, Minute Maid Orange Juice,** and **Knudsen Sour Cream.** Grind four tablespoons Quaker Oats in a blender or coffee grinder to make a fine powder. In a bowl, mix together two teaspoons Minute Maid Orange Juice, one teaspoon Knudsen Sour Cream, and one egg yolk. Stir in enough ground Quaker Oats to make a paste. Apply to your face, wait ten minutes, then rinse clean with warm water.

■ **Quaker Oats, Mott's Applesauce,** and **ReaLemon.** For oily skin, cook up one-half cup Quaker Oats (with water) according to the directions on the canister. When the oatmeal cools to the touch, mix with one-half cup Mott's Applesauce, one tablespoon ReaLemon lemon juice, and one egg white. Apply to your face, wait ten minutes, then wipe clean with a damp washcloth.

■ **Quaker Oats** and **SueBee Honey.** Mix up one cup warm oatmeal (with water) according to the directions on the canister, add enough honey to thicken, let cool to the touch, and then apply to your dry face. Wait ten minutes, then rinse with warm water. The warmth and the honey draw the oil from your skin, and the oatmeal absorbs it.

■ **R.W. Knudsen Black Cherry Juice** and **Quaker Oats.** Mix two tablespoons R.W. Knudsen Black Cherry Juice and one tablespoon Quaker Oats. Apply to your face, wait five minutes, then rinse clean. The malic acid in the cherry juice exfoliates dead skin cells and accelerates cell renewal.

■ **ReaLemon.** With a whisk, mix together two tablespoons Rea-Lemon lemon juice with one egg white, beating for three minutes. Apply the mixture to your face, let sit for a half hour, and then rinse clean with warm water and apply a moisturizer.

■ **Reddi-wip.** Use whipped cream as a facial mask to moisturize dry skin and give it a healthy glow. Apply Reddi-wip to your face, wait twenty minutes, then wash off with warm water, followed by cold water.

■ **SueBee Honey.** Mix one tablespoon SueBee Honey with one egg white, smooth over face and throat, and wait ten minutes. Rinse off this firming mask with warm water.

■ **SueBee Honey.** If you have oily skin, use a fork to mash nine strawberries into a pulp. Add three tablespoons SueBee honey and mix into a thick paste. Apply to your face, let sit for a few minutes, and wash off with warm water, followed by cold water.

■ **SueBee Honey, Carnation Evaporated Milk, Heinz Apple Cider Vinegar,** and **Gold Medal Flour.** Mix three tablespoons Sue-Bee Honey, one-half cup Carnation Evaporated Milk, and four tablespoons Heinz Apple Cider Vinegar in a bowl. Add enough Gold Medal Flour to make a thick paste. Apply as a face mask and let dry. Rinse off the mask with warm water, followed by cold water. The honey disinfects the skin and seals in moisture, the milk moisturizes, and the vinegar tightens the pores.

■ **SueBee Honey, Dannon Yogurt,** and **Carnation Nonfat Dry Milk.** Mix three tablespoons SueBee Honey, one tablespoon Dannon Plain Yogurt, and enough Carnation Nonfat Dry Milk to make a paste. Smooth over your face, wait fifteen minutes, and rinse clean with warm water, followed by cool water. Pat dry with a towel.

■ **SueBee Honey** and **International Collection Sweet Almond Oil.** Mix one teaspoon SueBee honey, one teaspoon International Collection Sweet Almond Oil, one teaspoon vitamin E oil, and one egg yolk until smooth. Spread the mixture over your face, let sit fifteen minutes, then rinse clean with warm water. Pat dry.

■ **Tidy Cats.** Mix two handfuls unused Tidy Cats Regular Clay with enough water to make a thick, muddy paste. Smear the mud over your face to create a deep cleansing mud mask, let set for twenty minutes, then rinse clean with water. The clay from the cat box filler detoxifies your skin by absorbing dirt and excess oil from the pores.

Immerse Yourself

■ Before applying a face mask, wash your face and pat dry with a towel to increase the effectiveness of the face mask.

■ Apply a facial mask to well-cleansed skin by smoothing it on evenly in upward strokes. Avoid areas around the eyes, nostrils, and the lips, but apply to the neck. Relax for ten to fifteen minutes, allowing the mask to dry, then rinse with warm water. For a deep-cleansing facial, use your fingertips to rub the dried mask away so you exfoliate the skin. Facial masks help clean pores, absorb oils, and give skin a radiant glow.

■ The 1957 movie *The Three Faces of Eve* stars Joanne Woodward as a schizophrenic patient with three distinctly different personalities: a mousy housewife, a party animal, and a sophisticated lady.

■ The Verabella salon in Beverly Hills offers a facial treatment called Fall on Your Face, consisting of a cranberry-apple scrub and a pumpkin-pie peel. A second facial treatment called Champagne and Caviar features a mask made from flat champagne mixed with powdered wheat germ and oatmeal, followed by a spongy sheet of collagen and caviar extract.

Feet

■ **Adolph's Original Unseasoned Tenderizer.** Add enough water to Adolph's Original Unseasoned Tenderizer to make a paste and rub the mixture into your feet to relax them. The enzymes in meat tenderizer numb the skin.

■ **Alberto VO5 Conditioning Hairdressing.** To soften your feet, coat them with Alberto VO5 Conditioning Hairdressing before going to bed and cover them with a pair of socks. In the morning, your feet will feel rejuvenated.

■ **Alka-Seltzer.** Add four Alka-Seltzer tablets to a basin of warm water and soak your tired feet in the alkaline solution for fifteen minutes (unless you are allergic to aspirin, a key ingredient in Alka-Seltzer).

■ **Arm & Hammer Baking Soda.** Dissolve three tablespoons Arm & Hammer Baking Soda in a basin of warm water and soak your achy feet in the solution for soothing relief.

■ **C&H Cane Sugar, Arm & Hammer Baking Soda, McCormick Poppy Seed,** and **ReaLemon.** Mix one-half cup C&H Cane Sugar, one tablespoon Arm & Hammer Baking Soda, one teaspoon McCormick Poppy Seed, and a few drops of ReaLemon lemon juice. Apply to your feet, scrub with a vegetable brush, and rinse clean.

■ **Carnation NonFat Dry Milk, Morton Salt,** and **Star Olive Oil.** Mix ten ounces Carnation Nonfat Dry Milk and twenty-five ounces warm water in a wide bowl. Soak your feet in the warm milky solution for ten minutes and then rinse clean. The lactic acids in the milk soften tough skin. In a bowl, mix one-half cup Morton Salt and one-third cup Star Olive Oil. Scrub your feet with the salt and olive oil mixture. Rinse clean with warm water, apply a moisturizer, and wear thick socks to seal in the softness.

■ **Carnation NonFat Dry Milk, Bigelow Plantation Mint Classic Tea Bags, McCormick Rosemary Leaves, McCormick Pure Peppermint Extract,** and **Saran Wrap.** Mix three ounces Carnation NonFat Dry Milk and eight ounces warm water in a wide bowl. Add the contents of one Bigelow Plantation Mint Classic Tea Bag, one teaspoon McCormick Rosemary Leaves, and one teaspoon McCormick Pure Peppermint Extract. Using a washcloth, apply the solution to your feet, wrap in Saran Wrap, wait five minutes, and rinse clean.

■ **Cool Whip.** Coat your feet with Cool Whip, wait fifteen minutes, then rinse clean. The coconut and palm kernel oils cool achy feet, moisturizing and softening the skin.

■ **Crisco All-Vegetable Shortening.** Massage your feet with a dab of Crisco All-Vegetable Shortening. Rub the soles of your feet with your thumbs and also concentrate between the toes.

■ **Dole Crushed Pineapple, Mott's Applesauce, ReaLemon, Ocean Spray Grapefruit Juice, McCormick Pure Anise Extract, Morton Salt,** and **Saran Wrap.** Mix together one-half cup Dole Crushed Pineapple, four tablespoons Mott's Applesauce, one teaspoon ReaLemon lemon juice, one-quarter cup Ocean Spray Grapefruit Juice, two teaspoons McCormick Pure Anise Extract, and one teaspoon Morton Salt. Massage the mixture into your feet. Wrap in Saran Wrap, wait thirty minutes, and rinse clean with warm water.

■ **Dr. Bronner's Peppermint Soap.** Rub a few drops of Dr. Bronner's Peppermint Soap into your feet to boost circulation.

■ **Epsom Salt** and **Lubriderm.** To soothe swollen ankles and tried feet, dissolve two tablespoons Epsom Salt in a basin of one quart warm water, soak your feet for ten minutes, then rinse clean with cool water, pat dry, and rub in Lubriderm to seal in the moisture.

■ **French's Mustard.** To soothe tired feet, fill a pan with two quarts warm water, mix in three tablespoons French's Mustard, and soak your feet in the luxurious mustard bath.

■ **Fruit of the Earth Aloe Vera Gel** and **McCormick Pure Peppermint Extract.** Mix two tablespoons Fruit of the Earth Aloe Vera Gel and one teaspoon McCormick Pure Peppermint Extract. Massage the mixture into your feet. The aloe vera cools and moisturizes the feet, and the peppermint stimulates circulation.

■ **Heinz White Vinegar.** To cool and dry your feet, use a cotton ball saturated with Heinz White Vinegar to swab your feet.

■ **Heinz White Vinegar.** Prevent toenail fungus from growing by soaking your toes in Heinz White Vinegar (or by saturating a Q-Tips cotton swab with vinegar and dabbing it around the toenail, underneath the toenail, and into the cuticle). Repeat daily until the infected toenail grows out and can be clipped away.

■ **Jell-O.** Following the directions on the box, make up three boxes of Jell-O of any flavor in a Rubbermaid container and let the gelatin solidify in the refrigerator. Soak your feet in the Jell-O for twenty minutes to deodorize your smelly feet.

■ **Kingsford's Corn Starch.** After taking a shower or bath, pat your feet dry and then powder your feet with Kingsford's Corn

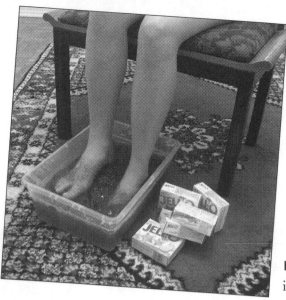

Starch, which absorbs moisture just like talcum powder.

■ **Listerine.** Cure toenail fungus by soaking your toes in Listerine four times daily for a couple of weeks. Listerine is an antiseptic that kills foot fungus.

■ **Listerine.** Soak your feet in Listerine for ten minutes to let the antiseptic solution kill any odor-causing bacteria. Rinse clean and pat dry.

■ **Morton Salt.** To deodorize smelly feet, dissolve one cup Morton Salt in one gallon warm water and soak your feet in the solution. Salt water dries the skin.

■ **Morton Kosher Salt, ReaLemon,** and **Star Olive Oil.** Mix together one-half cup Morton Kosher Salt, two tablespoons ReaLemon lemon juice, and two teaspoons Star Olive Oil. Massage the mixture into your feet, rinse clean with warm water, pat dry, and moisturize.

■ **Nestea.** Mix Nestea according to the directions in two quarts of warm water, soak your feet in the mixture, then rinse clean. The tannin in the tea tenderizes tired feet and dries the skin, bringing foot odor under control.

■ **Quaker Oats, Carnation Evaporated Milk,** and **SueBee Honey.** Mix one cup Quaker Oats, one-half cup Carnation Evaporated

Milk, and one-third cup SueBee Honey in a dish pan. Place your feet in the pan, coat them with the mixture by rubbing your feet back and forth, and let soak for twenty minutes. The mixture will leave your feet feeling smooth and moist.

■ **Quaker Oats** and **ReaLemon.** Add one cup Quaker Oats and two teaspoons ReaLemon lemon juice to a basin filled with warm water. Soak your feet for ten minutes, rubbing the oatmeal over your feet. The alpha-hydroxy acids in the lemon juice and scrubbing with the coarse oatmeal exfoliates dead skin, leaving your feet feeling smooth and soft.

■ **Scotch-Brite Heavy Duty Scrub Sponge.** To provide comfort for your feet when you walk, cut a Scotch-Brite Heavy Duty Scrub Sponge in half to make a cushion support to be inserted in your shoe.

■ **Smirnoff Vodka.** To cool down your feet, use a cotton ball saturated with Smirnoff Vodka to swab your feet. The alcohol in the vodka works like a liniment to cool and dry your feet.

■ **Tabasco Pepper Sauce.** Rub the hot sauce onto your feet. Tabasco Pepper Sauce, made from a type of pepper called Capsicum frutescens, contains the alkaloid capsaicin, which has been proven to numb pain when applied topically. Capsaicin enters nerves and temporarily depletes them of the neurotransmitter that sends pain signals to the brain. If you feel a burning sensation on the skin, apply a thin coat of Colgate Toothpaste over the dried Tabasco Pepper Sauce to relieve the irritation and possibly elevate the analgesia from the capsaicin. Do not apply Tabasco Pepper Sauce to an open wound.

■ **Vaseline Petroleum Jelly.** To moisturize and soften your feet, slather Vaseline Petroleum Jelly on your feet and cover with a pair of socks before going to bed. In the morning, your feet will feel like a million bucks.

■ **Vaseline Petroleum Jelly.** To avoid getting blisters from new shoes, apply a dab of Vaseline Petroleum Jelly over the areas of your skin that rub against the leather.

■ **Vicks VapoRub.** To soothe aching feet, apply a thick coat of Vicks VapoRub and cover with a pair of socks before going to bed. In the morning, your feet will be moisturized and rejuvenated.

■ **Vicks VapoRub.** Cure toenail fungus by applying a thick coat of Vicks VapoRub over the affected nail several times a day.

■ **Wesson Corn Oil.** Warm one-half cup Wesson Corn Oil in a microwave oven, let cool to the touch, and rub the warmed oil into your feet. Wrap in a damp, hot towel for ten minutes. Rinse clean and pat dry with a towel. The corn oil softens and moisturizes dry, achy feet.

■ **Wilson Tennis Balls.** Give yourself a relaxing foot massage by simply rolling your bare foot over a Wilson Tennis Ball for a few minutes.

Immerse Yourself

■ The average person walks approximately four miles every day or 115,000 miles over a lifetime. That's equivalent to walking around the world four times.

■ If your feet ache from being cooped up in tight shoes, walk around your house barefoot to stretch the muscles in your soles.

■ Soaking your feet in a hot immersion bath for four minutes, switching to a cold immersion bath for one minute, and repeating

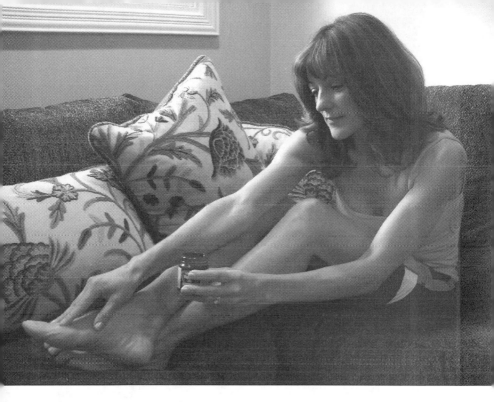

this routine for a total of thirty minutes boosts circulation to the feet. (If you have diabetes, avoid hot applications to the feet or legs.)

■ The best exercise for your feet is walking, which contributes to your general health by improving circulation, contributing to weight control, and promoting all-around well being.

■ In the New Testament, before the Last Supper, Jesus washes the feet of his disciples.

■ The Chinese practice of foot binding reportedly began in the court of a tenth century prince, whose favorite concubine wrapped her feet with silk ribbons to dance for him on her toes. For one thousand years, parents bound the feet of their daughters with tight strips of cloth to stunt the growth of their feet and reshape them into an erotic "lotus bud" form.

■ While other people claimed they never forgot a face, Dr. William Scholl, who at age twenty-two patented and launched the Foot-Eazer arch support, insisted that he never forgot a foot.

Hands

■ **C&H Cane Sugar** and **Johnson's Baby Oil.** Place one teaspoon C&H Cane Sugar in your palm, cover with Johnson's Baby Oil, rub your hands together, and then wash with soap. The abrasive sugar exfoliates dry skin.

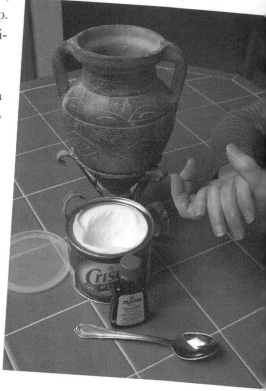

■ **Cheerios.** Using a blender, grind one cup Cheerios into a fine powder, then pour them into a large bowl. Rub the pulverized oats over your hands to exfoliate the dry skin. Wash your hands with cool water, dry well, then apply a moisturizing cream.

■ **Crisco All-Vegetable Shortening.** Soak your hands in warm water for five minutes, then seal in the moisture by coating your hands with a small dab of Crisco All-Vegetable Shortening.

■ **Johnson's Baby Powder.** Sprinkle Johnson's Baby Powder on your hands and rub into the skin to smooth rough hands.

■ **Johnson's Baby Powder.** Wearing rubber gloves while washing the dishes can irritate skin. Sprinkle Johnson's Baby Powder inside the gloves to reduce friction against the skin and to help the gloves slip on and off easily.

■ **Morton Salt** and **Johnson's Baby Oil.** To exfoliate dry skin from hands, mix Johnson's Baby Oil and Morton Salt to make an abrasive, moisturizing scrub.

■ **Neosporin.** To soothe dry hands, rub Neosporin antibiotic ointment into the skin as a hand cream.

■ **Playtex Living Gloves.** Before washing the dishes, apply skin cream to your hands, then put on a pair of Playtex Living Gloves. The heat from the warm water helps the skin cream penetrate your skin, deeply moisturizing your hands.

■ **Quaker Oats.** Blend one cup Quaker Oats into a fine powder and then rub the powdered oats over your hands to exfoliate the dry skin. Wash your hands with cool water, dry well, and then apply a moisturizing cream.

■ **Star Olive Oil, ReaLemon, SueBee Honey,** and **Ziploc Storage Bags.** Mix one-quarter cup Star Olive Oil, one tablespoon ReaLemon lemon juice, and one tablespoon SueBee Honey. Rub this lotion on over your hands and cover each hand with a Ziploc Storage Bag for twenty minutes. Rinse clean.

■ **Star Olive Oil** and **SueBee Honey.** Mix two teaspoons Star Olive Oil, two teaspoons SueBee Honey, and one drop geranium essential oil. Rub this lotion on your hands and wear cotton gloves or socks for thirty minutes.

■ **Vaseline Petroleum Jelly.** Before going to bed, rub Vaseline

Petroleum Jelly into your hands, put on a pair of cotton gloves (or wear a pair of cotton socks on your hands), and go to sleep. In the morning, your hands will be remarkably soft.

■ **Vaseline Petroleum Jelly** and **Ziploc Storage Bags.** Coat your hands with Vaseline Petroleum Jelly, slip them inside two Ziploc Storage Bags, wait fifteen minutes, then wash your hands with warm water.

■ **Wesson Corn Oil** and **Ziploc Storage Bags.** Massage Wesson Corn Oil into your hands, slip them inside two Ziploc Storage Bags, wait fifteen minutes, remove the excess oil with paper towels, then wash your hands with warm, soapy water.

Immerse Yourself

■ Humans are the only primates that do not have pigment in the palms of their hands.

■ On August 23, 1989, two million people held hands to form a human chain 370 miles long across Estonia, Latvia, and Lithuania.

■ 12.6 percent of all men are left-handed, compared to 9.9 percent of all women.

■ Dancing legend Fred Astaire had very large hands, which he disguised by curling his middle two fingers while dancing.

■ In 1964, the Beatle's hit single, "I Want to Hold Your Hand" reached Number One on all music charts in the United States.

■ On May 25, 1986, more than five million people held hands to form a human chain in various cities in an event called Hands Across America to raise money to fight hunger and homelessness. Enough people participated to form an unbroken chain that would have stretched 4,152 miles across the country from New York City's Battery Park to a pier in Long Beach, California.

Hydrotherapy

HOMEMADE FLOTATION TANK

■ **Epsom Salt.** Take a warm shower, washing your face, hair, and body. Fill the bathtub with warm water (around 84 degrees Fahrenheit) and mix six pounds Epsom Salt in the water (to increase the buoyancy of the water). Place earplugs in your ears to seal off extraneous sounds, turn off the lights, and relax in the tub for fifteen minutes, concentrating solely on how you're floating in the water. Allow yourself to be enveloped by a calming sense of weightlessness, letting physical tension and mental stress dissipate. Flotation tanks stimulate the body to produce endorphins—natural hormones that relief pain, lower blood pressure, and reduce stress. Epsom Salts baths, first used to treat shell-shocked soldiers during World War I, have a calming effect on the nerves.

HOMEMADE STEAM ROOM

■ **L'eggs Sheer Energy Panty Hose** and **Lipton Chamomile Tea Bags.** Cut off the foot from a clean, used pair of L'eggs Panty Hose, fill with the tea leaves from six Lipton Chamomile Tea Bags, and tie a knot in the nylon. Tie the sachet to the shower head, so it hangs under the stream of water. Close the bathroom door and windows and run the shower water on the hottest temperature for ten minutes, filling the bathroom with steam, scented by the herbs hanging in the sachet. Turn off the water and sit in the steam-filled room for an additional ten minutes. Steam opens the pores and prompts the body to perspire profusely, flushing out toxins and impurities. Take a warm shower, culminating with a short blast of cold water. Towel dry and drink water to avoid dehydration.

STEAM TREATMENTS

■ **Lipton Chamomile Tea Bags.** To clean pores and eliminate blackheads, fill a large bowl with boiling water and steep three

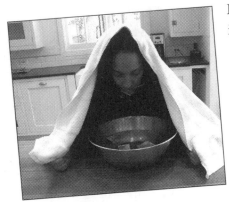

Lipton Chamomile Tea Bags. Wearing a towel over your head to form a tent over the bowl, hold your face close to the steaming tea for ten minutes. When the tea cools, dampen a washcloth with the tea and cleanse your face, rubbing in circles. Rinse clean with cool water and moisturize.

REHYDRATION

■ **C&H Cane Sugar, Morton Salt,** and **ReaLemon.** To make your own rehydration solution, mix three teaspoons C&H Cane Sugar, one teaspoon Morton salt, and two teaspoons ReaLemon lemon juice in a tall glass of water. Drink the entire solution to replace the glucose, minerals, and vitamin C being flushed out of your body.

■ **Gatorade.** Dehydration or profuse sweating causes a rise in body temperature, resulting in loss of appetite, headache, dizziness, and sometimes nausea and vomiting. Drinking Gatorade replaces electrolytes (the potassium and salt lost through perspiration) and prevents heat exhaustion.

Ice Packs

■ **Bounty Paper Towels.** To protect your skin when using an ice pack, wrap the ice pack in a sheet of a Bounty Paper Towel.

■ **Birds Eye Baby Peas.** Use a plastic bag of frozen Birds Eye Baby Peas as an ice pack. The sack of peas conforms to the contours of your body, and you can refreeze the peas for future ice-pack use. Be sure to label the bag for ice-pack use only. If you want to eat the peas, cook them after they thaw the first time, never after refreezing.

■ **Jell-O and Ziploc Freezer Bags.** Prepare Jell-O according to the directions on the box and let cool enough to pour into a Ziploc Freezer Bag until three-quarters full. Seal the bag shut securely and freeze, and you have a homemade, flexible ice pack that conforms to the shape of your body. When the Jell-O melts, simply refreeze.

■ **L'eggs Sheer Energy Panty Hose.** To protect the skin when using an ice pack, cut off one leg from a pair of L'eggs Sheer Energy Panty Hose, slip the ice pack inside, and tie a knot in the free end of the panty hose leg.

■ **Orville Redenbacher Gourmet Popping Corn** and **Ziploc**

Freezer Bags. Pour one cup unpopped kernels Orville Redenbacher Gourmet Popping Corn into a small Ziploc Freezer Bag and place in the freezer to make an ice pack that easily changes shape to match your body.

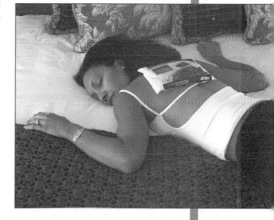

■ **Popsicle.** In a pinch, any flavor Popsicle works as an impromptu ice pack. Simply leave it in the wrapper and apply to the sore area of the skin.

■ **Smirnoff Vodka, Ziploc Freezer Bags,** and **McCormick Food Coloring.** Pour one-half cup Smirnoff Vodka and one-half cup water into a Ziploc Freezer Bag (add five drops of blue food coloring for easy identification) and freeze. The alcohol doesn't freeze, but the water does—giving you have a slushy, refreezable ice pack.

■ **Pampers.** If you are unable to take a shower or jump into a swimming pool to rehydrate your skin, saturate a Pampers diaper with water (the super-absorbent polymer flakes inside hold three hundred times their weight in liquid), wipe down your body, then wear it on your head to replenish your skin with moisture.

■ **Stayfree Maxi Pads.** If you don't have time to take a bath or shower, saturate a Stayfree Maxi Pad with water and use it as a washcloth to give yourself a sponge bath.

Immerse Yourself

■ Hydrotherapy consists of the use of ice, steam, and hot, tepid, and cold water in various ways to maintain health and promote healing.

■ Hydrotherapy treatments range from applying ice to a sprained ankle to soaking in a hot tub to soothe sore muscles.

■ Water hydrates the human body, cleans wounds, and prevents infection. Steam can open clogged sinuses. Ice packs can relieve swelling.

■ In the fourth century B.C.E., ancient Greek physician Hippocrates advocated the therapeutic effects of taking a bath.

■ Ancient Romans visited the bathhouse regularly as a part of their routine for good health and hygiene.

■ During the nineteenth century, Vincenz Priessnitz (1799-1851) and Father Sebastian Kneipp (1821-1897) established independent hydrotherapy centers in Germany, popularizing hydrotherapy.

■ At the end of the nineteenth century, hydrotherapy centers opened in the United States in Saratoga Springs, New York; Hot Springs, Arkansas; and Warm Springs, Georgia. President Franklin D. Roosevelt owned a house in Warm Springs, Georgia, where he frequented the mineral hot springs to ease the pain in his legs from his childhood battle with polio.

EPSOM SALT

It may look like ordinary table salt, but Epsom Salt is actually magnesium sulfate in crystal form. The pure mineral compound is named after the springs in Epsom, England, where it was first mined during William Shakespeare's day.

Magnesium, the second-most abundant element in human cells, helps to regulate the activity of more than 325 enzymes and performs a vital role in coordinating muscle control, electrical impulses, energy production, and the elimination of harmful toxins.

According to the National Academy of Sciences, most Americans are magnesium deficient, and this deficiency causes heart disease, stroke, osteoporosis, arthritis and joint pain, digestive maladies and stress-related illnesses, chronic fatigue, and a many other ailments.

The human body can absorb Epsom Salt, dissolved in a bath, through the skin, replenishing the body's levels of magnesium. Soaking in an Epsom Salt bath also relieves stress by raising the body's level of serotonin, lowering the affects of adrenaline, helping to regulate the electrical impulses in the nerves, and lowering blood pressure.

■ In 1900, Dr. J. H. Kellogg, the brother of the founder of the Kellogg cereal company, published his book *Rational Hydrotherapy*, documenting his research experiments on the therapeutic effects of water.

■ Water stores and transmits cold and heat. Ice packs and cold compresses constrict blood vessels, numb nerves, and slow respiration. Hot baths and hot compresses cause blood vessels to dilate, increasing circulation to the area being treated.

■ Rubbing the skin vigorously in a circular motion with a towel, washcloth, or mitten dipped in cold water increases circulation, strengthens the immune system, and relieves fatigue.

■ Wearing a pair of wet socks covered by a pair of dry wool socks encourages sleep and relaxation. The body's heat warms the wet socks, creating a soothing warmth in the affected area.

■ Alternating heat and cold hydrotherapies dramatically stimulates local circulation. For example, soaking your legs in a hot immersion bath for four minutes, switching to a cold immersion bath for one minute, and repeating this routine for a total of thirty minutes can produce a 95 percent increase in local blood flow. (If you have diabetes, avoid hot applications to the feet or legs.)

■ Alternating hot and cold soaks relieves swelling in the feet and legs and can be used to relieve head and chest congestion and menstrual cramps (by diverting blood away from the affected areas).

■ Cold baths or showers relieve fever and fatigue. Hot baths or showers relieve joint pain, constipation, and respiratory ailments. (Avoid hot baths if you have diabetes, multiple sclerosis, high or low blood pressure, or if you are pregnant.)

■ Immersing yourself up to the neck in bathwater slightly cooler than body temperature for twenty minutes relieves insomnia, stress, anxiety, and menopausal hot flashes. (Avoid cold applications if you have Raynaud's disease.)

■ The average person drinks 8,000 gallons of water during his or her lifetime.

■ Gatorade rehydrates the body 30 percent faster than water.

■ When you feel thirsty, you are already in the early stages of dehydration.

■ Affusion—pouring water over parts of the body—stimulates the body and awakens the mind.

■ A hot shower stimulates circulation and relives aching muscles, and switching the water temperature to give yourself short bursts of cold water invigorates both body and mind.

■ Russian cosmonaut Valery Polyakov, who lived aboard the *Mir* Space Station for 437 days, used wet towels to wash his skin and hair.

Lips & Mouth

LIPS

■ **Alberto VO5 Conditioning Hairdressing.** To soothe chapped lips, rub in a dab of Alberto VO5 Hairdressing.

■ **Bag Balm.** Keep chapped lips moist and happy by rubbing on a dab of Bag Balm, the salve created to relieve cracking in cow udders.

■ **Balmex.** Apply a dab of Balmex, the diaper rash ointment that contains aloe and zinc oxide, to your lips to keep them moisturized and nourished, providing a barrier against wetness.

■ **ChapStick.** To make your lips appear sensuous and plump, simply apply a dab of cherry-flavored ChapStick in the center of your lips.

■ **ChapStick** and **Oral-B Toothbrush.** Exfoliate chapped lips by applying mint-flavored ChapStick to your lips and then brushing your lips gently with a clean, used Oral-B Toothbrush.

■ **Coppertone.** A dab of Coppertone will keep lips moist and healthy while simultaneously preventing the ultraviolet rays from the sun from drying out the lips.

■ **Crisco All-Vegetable Shortening.** Moisturize chapped lips with a dab of Crisco All-Vegetable Shortening.

■ **Crisco All-Vegetable Shortening** and **Kool-Aid.** To make your own lip gloss, place three tablespoons Crisco All-Vegetable Shortening in a ceramic coffee cup and heat in a microwave oven for one minute (or until the shortening liquefies). Empty a packet of your favorite flavor Kool-Aid into the cup of melted shortening and stir well until dissolved. Carefully pour the colored liquid into a clean, empty 35mm Kodak Film canister, cap tightly, and refrigerate overnight. In the morning, you've got tasty homemade lip gloss that moisturizes chapped lips.

■ **Dannon Yogurt** and **Quaker Oats.** Mix one teaspoon Dannon Plain Yogurt and one-half teaspoon Quaker Oats. Massage the mixture into your lips with your fingertips and rinse clean with water.

■ **Gatorade.** Help heal chapped lips by drinking Gatorade. Keeping your body well hydrated keeps your lips naturally moist, giving your chapped lips the moisture they need to heal themselves.

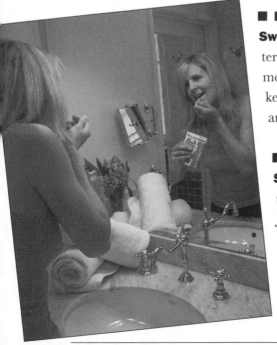

■ **International Collection Sweet Almond Oil.** Apply International Collection Sweet Almond Oil around the mouth to keep your lips supple and soften any lines.

■ **Jell-O** and **Q-Tips Cotton Swabs.** Moisten a Q-Tips Cotton Swab with water, dip it into Jell-O powder (any flavor and color you wish), and apply it to your lips. Wait five minutes and then lick off the powder, leaving your lips with an accent of flavorful color.

■ **Johnson's Baby Oil.** Use a drop of Johnson's Baby Oil to moisturize your chapped lips. (Just be sure to stay out of the sun. Mineral oil makes your lips more susceptible to sunburn, which can chap your lips further.)

■ **Lipton Tea Bags.** To reduce swollen lips, dampen a Lipton Tea Bag with warm water and press over clean lips for five minutes. The tannic acid in the tea retains moisture and keeps lips smooth and taut.

■ **Maybelline MoistureWhip Lipstick.** To protect your lips from the sun's visible light, wear an opaque lipstick like Maybelline Moisture Whip Lipstick.

■ **McCormick Mint Extract.** To plump up your lips, mix a drop of McCormick Mint Extract with your lip gloss. Mint stimulates circulation, swelling lips briefly.

■ **Noxzema.** Applying a dab of Noxzema to chapped lips helps soothe and heal them. The cream moisturizes your lips, and the bitter taste will prevent you from licking your lips further.

■ **Oral-B Toothbrush.** Use a clean Oral-B Toothbrush to exfoliate chapped lips by brushing them gently in a circular motion. Brushing your lips will also make them swell temporarily, making your lips appear plump and full.

■ **SueBee Honey.** Mix one tablespoon SueBee Honey and one teaspoon water and melt the mixture in a microwave oven for approximately twenty seconds. Let cool, then apply to chapped lips.

■ **Vaseline Petroleum Jelly.** Applying a dab of Vaseline Petroleum Jelly to your lips moisturizes and protects your lips just like ChapStick.

■ **Vaseline Petroleum Jelly.** Adding a dab of Vaseline Petroleum Jelly on top of regular lipstick creates an attractive gloss.

■ **Vaseline Petroleum Jelly** and **McCormick Pure Peppermint Extract.** Mix one tablespoon Vaseline and three drops McCormick Pure Peppermint Extract to make a mint-flavored lip gloss.

MOUTH

■ **Alka-Seltzer.** Dissolve two Alka-Seltzer tablets in a glass of warm water and swish the fizzy solution through your mouth as a mouthwash (unless you are allergic to aspirin, a key ingredient in Alka-Seltzer). The sodium bicarbonate in the Alka-Seltzer lowers the pH level in your mouth, killing odor-producing bacteria.

■ **Arm & Hammer Baking Soda.** Dissolve two teaspoons Arm & Hammer Baking Soda in a glass of warm water and use the solution as a mouthwash. The sodium bicarbonate solution raises the acid level in your mouth, inhibiting bacteria from producing smelly sulfur compounds.

■ **Bigelow Plantation Mint Classic Tea Bags.** Brew a strong cup of Bigelow Plantation Mint Classic Tea and drink it, swishing the tea around your mouth. Or let the mint tea cool and gargle.

■ **Country Time Lemonade.** Put one teaspoon Country Time Lemonade powdered drink mix in your mouth, swish around, and swallow. The citric acid stimulates saliva production, hinders the odor-producing enzymes in your mouth, and makes your breath lemon fresh.

■ **Dr. Bronner's Peppermint Soap.** Mix two drops of Dr. Bronner's Peppermint Soap and one cup water, rinse your mouth with the solution, and spit out. Dr. Bronner's Peppermint Soap, made from 100 percent vegetable oil, will kill the bacteria that produce foul-smelling sulfur compounds in your mouth.

■ **Heinz Apple Cider Vinegar.** Make a potent mouthwash by mixing equal parts Heinz Apple Cider Vinegar and water in a drinking glass. The acetic acid in the vinegar lowers the pH level in your mouth, killing odor-producing bacteria.

■ **Hydrogen Peroxide.** Mix equal parts hydrogen peroxide (three percent solution) and water, rinse your mouth with the solution for thirty seconds, and spit out. The hydrogen peroxide kills the bacteria that generate odors in your mouth.

■ **Lipton Tea Bags.** According to scientists at the College of Dentistry at the University of Illinois in Chicago, compounds in tea, known as polyphenols, can halt the growth of sulphur-producing bacteria in the mouth and inhibit the enzyme that catalyzes the formation of smelly hydrogen sulphide. To fight bad breath, drink a cup of tea brewed with a Lipton Tea Bag, or let the tea cool and use as a mouthwash.

■ **MasterCard.** Scrape off the white or yellow coating on your tongue with the edge of a clean credit card. Scraping your tongue removes the habitat that enables odor-producing bacteria to breed in your mouth.

■ **McCormick Ground Cinnamon, Smirnoff Vodka,** and **Mr. Coffee Filters.** Mix nine tablespoons McCormick Ground Cin namon, one cup Smirnoff Vodka, and one cup water. Seal in an airtight container and let sit for two weeks, shaking the contents twice a day. Strain the liquid through a Mr. Coffee Filter. To use, mix one tablespoon of the solution in a glass of warm water and rinse your mouth with the tangy mouthwash.

■ **McCormick Fennel Seed.** Chewing a few fennel seeds destroys the bacteria in your mouth that cause bad breath.

■ **McCormick Whole Cloves** and **McCormick Cinnamon Sticks.** Steep a few cloves with a cinnamon stick in a tea cup filled with boiling water. Let cool and gargle with this natural mouthwash.

■ **McCormick Pure Peppermint Extract.** Mix one tablespoon McCormick Pure Peppermint Extract in one cup water and gargle with the mixture.

■ **ReaLemon.** Add a few drops of ReaLemon lemon juice to a glass of warm water, swish the lemony solution around your mouth around, and swallow. The citric acid alters the pH level in your mouth, killing bacteria and leaving your breath lemon fresh.

■ **Tang.** Put one teaspoon of Tang powdered drink mix in your mouth, swish around, and swallow. The citric acid in Tang prompts saliva production, inhibits the odor-producing enzymes in your mouth, and freshens your breath.

TEETH

■ **Arm & Hammer Baking Soda.** Dip a wet toothbrush into Arm & Hammer Baking Soda to coat the bristles with a thick layer of powder and brush your teeth, concentrating along the gum line. The sodium bicarbonate lowers the pH level in your mouth (neutralizing odor-producing bacteria) and deodorizes your mouth, and the abrasive granules gently polish your teeth.

■ **Dentyne.** Unable to brush your teeth after a meal? Chewing a piece of Dentyne sugarless gum for twenty minutes causes your mouth to salivate, washing your teeth and neutralizing the acid in the plaque.

■ **Easy Cheese.** Studies conducted by the Dow Institute for Dental Studies at the University of Iowa show that five grams of cheddar cheese (less than an ounce), when eaten before meals, helps maintain a pH level in the mouth that inhibits the acid production of plaque.

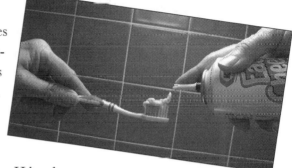

■ **Fruit of the Earth Aloe Vera Gel.** If your gums bleed from inadequate brushing, squeeze a dab of Fruit of the Earth Aloe Vera Gel on a toothbrush and brush your gums to help them heal and to reduce plaque.

■ **Lipton Tea Bags.** According to scientists at the College of Dentistry at the University of Illinois in Chicago, black tea suppresses the growth of bacteria in dental plaque, reduces plaque formation, and inhibits production of acids that cause tooth decay. Drink a cup of tea brewed with a Lipton Tea Bag, or let the tea cool and as a mouthwash.

■ **Listerine.** Rinsing your mouth with Listerine helps prevent and reduce supragingival plaque accumulation and gingivitis when used in a conscientiously applied program of oral hygiene and regular professional care.

■ **McCormick Food Coloring.** To spot plaque on your teeth, put ten drops of red food coloring in a glass, add one teaspoon water, and swirl well. Pour the red solution into your mouth, swish it around well, then spit out. Fill the glass with clean water and rinse your mouth well. The remaining red stains on your teeth are plaque. Brush these areas well.

■ **Ocean Spray Cranberry Juice Cocktail.** Drinking cranberry juice, according to scientists at Tel Aviv University School of Dental Medicine in Israel, prevents plaque-forming bacteria from adhering to teeth, thwarting gingivitis and gum disease.

Immerse Yourself

■ Lips, lacking sweat glands and having few sebaceous glands, are naturally protected by saliva.

■ When buying lipstick, bite your lips for thirty seconds and choose a shade of lipstick that matches that color (or the color of the inside of your lower lip).

■ When brushing your teeth, do not wet the toothpaste under running water. Toothpaste straight from the tube on a toothbrush and used dry works better and requires less product.

■ Drinking water prevents bad breath. Otherwise, your mouth doesn't produce enough saliva to dissolve gases containing sulfur.

■ Test the color of lipstick on your fingertips, where the texture and color of the skin most closely matches your lips.

■ Rather than buying a dozen shades of lipstick, you can mix your own lipstick colors by dipping a paint brush into various lipstick tubes and mixing the colors on a sheet of Reynolds Cut-Rite Wax Paper.

■ Ancient Greek courtesans (mistresses of wealthy men) perfumed their breath with an aromatic oil that they swished around their mouths and then spit out.

Manicures & Pedicures

■ Alberto VO5 Conditioning Hairdressing. To soften dry cuticles, rub a dab of Alberto VO5 Conditioning Hairdressing into the cuticle of each finger. The five vital organic ingredients in the hairdressing moisturize the cuticle.

■ Alberto VO5 Conditioning Hairdressing. Apply a dab of Alberto VO5 Conditioning Hairdressing to painted fingernails and buff with a cotton ball to rejuvenate the shine of the nail polish and strengthen the nails, preventing chips and breaks.

■ Aqua Net Hair Spray. If you don't have any nail polish remover, you can remove nail polish by spraying your nails with Aqua Net Hair Spray. The acetone in the hair spray dissolves nail polish.

■ Arm & Hammer Baking Soda and **Oral-B Toothbrush.** Whiten fingernails by adding three tablespoons Arm & Hammer Baking soda to one-half cup warm water. Soak your nails in the solution for fifteen minutes. Then softly brush across each nail with a clean, used Oral-B toothbrush (or a regular nailbrush).

■ Bag Balm. To moisturize cuticles and soften brittle nails, massage Bag Balm around your fingernails before going to bed, put on a pair of white cotton gloves or socks, and go to sleep. By morning your cuticles will be soft and healthy.

■ **Bounce.** To remove nail polish without the aid of nail polish remover, rub a Bounce dryer sheet over your fingernails.

■ **ChapStick.** Condition dry, cracked cuticles by rubbing on ChapStick Lip Balm. Also, applying ChapStick to your fingernails before applying an alpha hydroxy lotion to your hands prevents the acids from weakening, breaking, and splitting your nails.

■ **ChapStick.** If you want to make your nails appear polished, apply a dab of ChapStick to each nail and buff.

■ **Clorox Bleach.** To remove nail polish stains, mix four teaspoons Clorox Bleach and one cup warm water and soak nails in the mixture for fifteen minutes.

■ **Colgate Toothpaste.** Use a dab of Colgate Regular Flavor Toothpaste on a toothbrush to gently scrub away excess cuticle, smooth rough edges, or to clean ink or dried glue from your nails.

■ **Conair Pro Styler 1600.** Dry nail polish on your fingernails by blowing them with warm air from a Conair Pro Styler 1600.

■ **Coppertone.** To soften and moisturize brittle fingernails, warm three teaspoons Coppertone in the microwave and, when cool to the touch, apply to your fingernails as a hot oil treatment.

■ **Coppertone.** Wearing sunscreen over polished fingernails prevents the color from fading.

■ **Crisco All-Vegetable Shortening.** Moisturize cuticles by applying a thin coat of Crisco All-Vegetable Shortening.

■ **Crisco All-Vegetable Shortening, Saran Wrap,** and **Scotch Transparent Tape.** To treat a hangnail, apply a dab of Crisco

All-Vegetable Shortening on the affected area before going to bed, wrap the fingertip with a piece of Saran Wrap, and secure in place with Scotch Transparent Tape. The plastic wrap confines the moisture overnight, softening the cuticle by morning so the hangnail can be easily removed.

■ **Dickinson's Witch Hazel.** Before applying nail polish, use a cotton ball to dab your fingernails with Dickinson's Witch Hazel to prevent bubbling.

■ **Dole Crushed Pineapple, Heinz Apple Cider Vinegar, Wesson Corn Oil, SueBee Honey,** and **Saran Wrap.** Mix one-quarter cup Dole Crushed Pineapple, one teaspoon Heinz Apple Cider Vinegar, one teaspoon Wesson Corn Oil, one tablespoon SueBee Honey, and one egg yolk. Apply the mixture to your hands, focusing on the cuticles. Wrap your hands in Saran Wrap, wait fifteen minutes, remove the plastic wrap, and rinse with warm water.

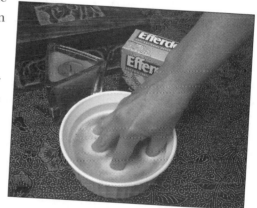

■ **Efferdent.** To whiten yellowed fingernails, dissolve two Efferdent tablets in a bowl of water and then soak your fingernails in the denture cleansing solution for five minutes.

■ **Forster Toothpicks.** In a pinch, you can use a Forster Toothpick as a manicure tool to clean dirt from under fingernails.

■ **Forster Toothpicks** and **Band-Aid Bandages.** After softening the nail and skin around an ingrown toenail and sterilizing the area with an antiseptic, use a Forster Toothpick to lift the sharp

How to Give Yourself a Manicure

■ Before giving yourself a manicure, remove any old nail polish from your nails (with Cutex Nail Polish Remover), wash your hands with soap and water, and, if necessary, clean any dirt from under your nails with a nail file.

■ Decide upon a shape for your nails. Petite hands and fingers look best with almond-shaped nails; short and stocky fingers look best with squoval-shaped nails (squared-off oval); heavy-set hands (and fingers with wide nail beds) look best with squared-off ends.) You can also match the shape of the free edge to the shape of the cuticle.

■ Before soaking your nails, shape them by using long gentle strokes in a single direction with an emery board (not a see-sawing stroke, which causes the keratin fibers to separate). Start at the outer corner of each nail, holding emery board at a 45 to 90 degree angle against the edge of the nail, and move toward the center, repeating until you achieve the desired shape. Then repeat on the opposite edge of the nail.

■ Shaping your fingernails so that the nail extends only slightly beyond the fingertip reduces the chances of breaking the nail.

■ After shaping your nails, soak them in a bowl of warm water for two minutes and then pat dry with a towel.

■ Rub some cuticle cream or oil on your cuticles and massage into the nail bed to soften them and then use an orange stick to gently push the cuticles back.

edge of the nail away form the skin. Insert a small piece of gauze or cotton under the tail, then cover with a Band-Aid Bandage to allow the nail to grow out. Change the dressing daily.

■ **Heinz White Vinegar.** Soften cuticles by soaking your fingertips or toes in small bowl filled with Heinz White Vinegar for five minutes. Or wrap your feet in a towel saturated with vinegar. Also,

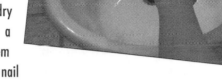

■ Unless you're going to color your nails, apply a rich moisturizer into your hands, massaging well.

■ Before coloring your nails, let them air dry thoroughly or use a blow-dryer to dry them fully. Do not apply nail polish to wet nails, otherwise the nail polish will peel off.

■ Before applying nail polish, buff your nails lightly with a white block buffer or an extra fine emery board (to smoothen the ridges and gently roughen the surface so the polish will adhere better).

■ Apply a thin base coat of nail polish and let dry until just slightly tacky.

■ Apply a thin coat of colored polish with three or four brush strokes. Visible brush marks on the nail will dry into an even coat. Let the polish dry completely and then apply a second thin coat and, if necessary, a third thin coat (after the second coat has dried completely).

■ Remove polish from your skin with a cotton pad dipped in nail polish remover or take a hot shower the following morning, allowing the steam to loosen the polish from your skin.

■ Apply a thin coat of topcoat or sealant and let it dry thoroughly. You can renew the topcoat every two to three days.

nail polish will adhere longer to fingernails that have been soaked in vinegar.

■ **Heinz White Vinegar.** Remove nail polish stains by soaking your fingernails in Heinz White Vinegar for ten minutes.

■ **Heinz White Vinegar** and **Q-Tips Cotton Swabs.** Prevent fingernail biting by using a Q-Tips Cotton Swab to paint your fingernails with a quick dab of Heinz White Vinegar. Let dry. Should you absentmindedly put your fingernails in your mouth, the tart taste will quickly get your attention, reminding you to stop biting your nails.

■ **Hydrogen Peroxide.** Whiten yellow fingernails by rubbing them with a cotton ball dampened with hydrogen peroxide.

■ **Jell-O** and **Q-Tips Cotton Swabs.** Strengthen your fingernails by mixing your favorite flavor of Jell-O powder with enough water to make a paste. Use a Q-Tips Cotton Swab to paint the colorful solution on your fingernails. The gelatin bolsters the nails, helping them grow longer and stronger. The richer Jell-O colors also tint your nails and give them a pleasant fruit-flavored bouquet.

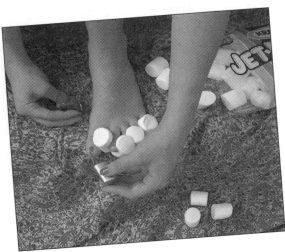

■ **Jet-Puffed Marshmallows.** If you do not have toenail separators, place a Jet-Puffed Marshmallow between each toe before painting your toenails with polish.

■ **Johnson's Baby Oil.** Rejuvenate brittle fingernails by warming a few tablespoons Johnson's Baby Oil in a microwave oven, letting it cool to the touch, and then soaking your nails in the warm oil for ten minutes.

■ **Kingsford's Corn Starch.** After taking a shower or bath, pat your feet dry and then powder your feet with Kingsford's Corn Starch, which absorbs moisture just like talcum powder.

MADGE THE MANICURIST

Beginning in 1966, the Colgate-Palmolive Company ran a series of highly successful television commercials starring a wisecracking manicurist named Madge. Working at the fictitious Salon East Beauty Parlor, Madge pre-soaked her customer's fingernails in Palmolive's green dishwashing detergent. She advised her clients to avoid dishpan hands by washing their dishes at home with Palmolive, which "softens hands while you do the dishes." When the customer expressed disbelief at Palmolive's curative powers, Madge replied with her catchphrase, "You're soaking in it." Popular worldwide, the Madge character was called Françoise in France, Tilly in Germany, and Marissa in Finland.

Actress Jan Miner played the part of Madge for twenty-seven years—until Colgate-Palmolive stopped running the commercials in 1992. Born in Boston in 1917, Miner trained as an actor with Lee Strasberg, costarred on the syndicated radio detective drama *Boston Blackie*, and on television, played Ann Williams on *Crime Photographer* and appeared as a regular on *Robert Montgomery Presents*. On the silver screen, Miner played Lenny Bruce's mother in the movie *Lenny*. She died in 2004 at the age of 86.

■ **Krazy Glue.** Fix a broken fingernail with a small drop of Krazy Glue, hold the nail in place for a few seconds, let dry, and then coat with the nail polish of your choice.

■ **Lipton Tea Bags** and **Maybelline Clear Nail Polish.** If you break a fingernail, cut a piece of gauze paper from a Lipton Tea Bag the size of the nail, coat the broken nail with Maybelline Crystal Clear Nail Polish, press the gauze paper over the wet nail polish, let dry, then paint over the gauze paper with nail polish.

■ **Lubriderm.** To avoid getting hangnails, moisturize your cuticles daily with Lubriderm to keep the flesh adjoining your nails supple.

■ **Lubriderm.** Applying Lubriderm to your hands and fingernails every day helps to maintain a manicure.

■ **MasterCard.** The corner of a MasterCard works as a manicure tool to clean under your fingernails.

■ **Miracle Whip.** To fortify your fingernails, coat them with Miracle Whip, wait five minutes, then wash clean.

■ **Mr. Coffee Filters** and **Krazy Glue.** To make nail wraps, cut a piece of a Mr. Coffee Filter to match the size of your fingernail and adhere it to the nail with a drop of Krazy Glue.

■ **Morton Salt** and **ReaLime.** Whiten yellowing fingernails by mixing one teaspoon Morton Salt and two teaspoons ReaLime lime juice in a bowl of warm water. Soak your fingernails for ten minutes.

■ **Noxzema.** Soften fingernails by warming Noxzema in the microwave and using it as a hot oil treatment.

■ **Orajel.** If you're suffering from an ingrown toenail, apply Orajel to numb the tissue around the nail so you can work on it.

■ **Oral-B Toothbrush.** If you do not have a nailbrush, dip a clean, used Oral-B Toothbrush in soapy water to clean fingernails gently and effectively.

■ **Palmolive Dishwashing Liquid.** To soften your cuticles, fill a bowl with warm water containing a tablespoon of Palmolive Dishwashing Liquid, mix well, and immerse your hands in the liquid for two minutes. Rinse clean with warm water and pat dry.

■ **Pam Cooking Spray.** Moisturize cuticles by spraying them with a thin coat of Pam Cooking Spray and then massaging the oil into the cuticle area.

■ **Pam Cooking Spray.** After painting your nails, spray with Pam Cooking Spray to dry the nail polish.

■ **ReaLemon, Heinz White Vinegar,** and **Oral-B Toothbrush.** Revitalize brittle fingernails, soften stiff cuticles, and whiten yellowed fingernails by soaking your fingers for ten minutes in a mixture of equal parts ReaLemon lemon juice and Heinz White Vinegar. Use a clean, used Oral-B Toothbrush (or a regular nailbrush) to brush the mixture over your fingernails. Rinse clean. The citric acid bleaches fingernails naturally.

■ **ReaLemon** and **Q-Tips Cotton Swabs.** To stop yourself from biting your fingernails, use a Q-Tips Cotton Swab to paint your fingernails with ReaLemon lemon juice. Let dry. Any time you absentmindedly put your fingers in your mouth, you'll get a tart reminder to break the habit.

■ **Skin-So-Soft.** Make your cuticles oh-so-soft by soaking your fingernails for fifteen minutes in one cup warm water to which two capfuls Skin-So-Soft have been added.

■ **Star Olive Oil.** Pour one-quarter cup Star Olive Oil in a bowl, warm in a microwave oven, and when cool to the touch, soak your fingertips in the oil for five minutes to condition the cuticles. Or apply warmed Star Olive Oil to your hands before bedtime, massage into the skin thoroughly, and wear a pair of thin plastic gloves to bed. In the morning, massage your hands, wipe away the excess oil with a tissue, rinse your hands, and pat dry with a towel.

How to Give Yourself a Pedicure

■ Use a cotton pad soaked with nail-polish remover to clean off old polish.

■ Fold a bath towel into a square and place it at the bottom of a clean, wide bucket. Fill the bucket with hot water and place it in front of a chair. Add one-half cup Epsom Salt and soak your feet in the solution for five minutes. Use a body rub or scrub (see page 102) to gently exfoliate dead skin. Use a pumice stone or a foot file to exfoliate the heels, ankles, and calluses. Pat feet dry with a towel.

■ If you have hard, cracking toenails or dry cuticles, soak them in small bowl of warm Star Olive Oil for five minutes.

■ Cut your toenails straight across with nail clippers or nail scissors (to avoid ingrown toenails). Use a nail file to smooth the edges.

■ Apply cuticle cream to each toenail and massage well into the nail bed for a minute, then gently push back the cuticles with an orange stick.

■ Apply moisturizer, massaging it into your feet and heels.

■ If you intend to apply nail polish, wash the moisturizer off your toenails with soap and water and let them dry thoroughly.

■ Before applying nail polish, buff your nails lightly with a white block buffer or an extra fine emery board (to smoothen the ridges and gently roughen the surface so the polish will adhere better).

■ **Star Olive Oil.** Mash a half-ripe avocado and mix with one teaspoon Star Olive Oil. Massage the mixture into cuticles, wait fifteen minutes, and rinse clean. Avocado oil is a rich moisturizer.

■ **Star Olive Oil.** Revitalize the shine of your polished fingernails by rubbing a drop of Star Olive Oil over each nail.

■ **Stayfree Ultra Thin Maxi Pads.** Stayfree Ultra Thin Maxi

- Create space between toes with a separator.
- Apply a thin base coat of nail polish and let dry until just slightly tacky.
- Apply a thin coat of colored polish with three or four brush strokes. Visible brush marks on the nail will dry into an even coat. Let the polish dry completely, then apply a second thin coat and, if necessary, a third thin coat (after the second coat has dried completely).

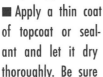

- Apply a thin coat of topcoat or sealant and let it dry thoroughly. Be sure to wait at least five minutes before applying the topcoat to avoid chipping.
- Use a Q-Tips Cotton Swab moistened with Cutex Nail Polish Remover to remove any polish from your skin.
- Allow the nail polish to dry for several hours before putting on shoes.
- To prevent the nail polish from chipping, apply a thin coat of top coat every three days.

Pads make excellent shoe insert pads. Not only are they the perfect size, but they are also available with deodorant—killing two birds with one stone.

■ **Tabasco Pepper Sauce** and **Q-Tips Cotton Swabs.** To stop yourself from biting your fingernails, use a Q-Tips Cotton Swab to dab your fingernails with Tabasco Pepper Sauce. Let dry. Should your fingernails unconsciously wander up to your lips, the zesty tang will quickly jolt your attention, reminding you to correct your behavior.

■ **Vaseline Petroleum Jelly.** To moisturize hardened cuticles, massage Vaseline Petroleum Jelly into the skin around your fingernails before going to bed, and wear a pair of white cotton gloves (or a pair of cotton socks on your hands) to sleep. In the morning, your cuticles will be supple once again.

■ **Vaseline Petroleum Jelly.** Prevent the cap from getting sealed shut on a nail polish bottle by rubbing a thin coat of Vaseline Petroleum Jelly around the spiral groves in the rim of the bottle.

■ **Wesson Corn Oil.** Moisturize your nails and cuticles by soaking them in warm Wesson Corn Oil and then massaging the oil into your fingers.

Immerse Yourself

■ Store nail polish in the refrigerator to prevent the polish from thickening through evaporation.

■ Regular nail polish lasts three times longer when painted on fingernails than quick-drying nail polish.

■ Do not shake bottles of nail polish, which adds air bubbles. Instead, roll the bottle upright between your palms.

■ Dipping your painted fingernails in ice water for fifteen seconds sets the color.

■ Extend the life of a bottle of nail polish by adding polish thinner (not nail polish remover).

■ Regular foot and nail care helps ward off ingrown toenails, calluses, foot cracks, and infections.

■ Toenails are made from dead skin cells called keratin, the same hard protein that forms hair.

Massage

■ **Adolph's Meat Tenderizer.** Mix one tablespoon Adolph's Meat Tenderizer with enough water to make a paste, then rub the mixture into your back as a liniment to soothe sore muscles.

■ **Alka-Seltzer.** Dissolve six Alka-Seltzer tablets in a bathtub filled with warm water and soak in the tub for fifteen minutes to relax kinks and stiffness in your muscles. For more ways to make a soothing bath, see page 6.

■ **Ban Roll-on Deodorant, Dawn Dishwashing Liquid,** and **Therapeutic Mineral Ice.** Pry the top off a used, empty canister of Ban Roll-on Deodorant and use a few drops of Dawn Dishwashing Liquid and running water to wash out the bottle, roller ball, and lid. Fill the canister with Therapeutic Mineral Ice, replace the roller, and rub on achy muscles. The canister delivers the Mineral Ice with the benefit of a massage—without getting any hot salve on your hands.

■ **BenGay.** Rub a small dab of BenGay into your forehead, temples, and the back of your neck. The heat from the salve will gently soothe tired muscles, and the heartening aroma of menthol will invigorate and stimulate your being.

■ **Castor Oil.** This natural emollient—first used as a skin softener throughout Mesopotamia and ancient Egypt—makes an excellent massage oil. If desired, you can scent castor oil with a few drops of McCormick Mint Extract, McCormick Pure Anise Extract, McCormick Pure Lemon Extract, McCormick Pure Orange Extract,

McCormick Pure Peppermint Extract, or McCormick Pure Vanilla Extract (or the appropriate pure essential oils listed on the chart on page 5).

■ **Coppertone.** Made with aloe extract, palm kernel oil, and jojoba oil, Coppertone sunscreen doubles as a terrific massage oil that just so happens to protect skin from UVA and UVB rays.

■ **Dynasty Sesame Seed Oil.** For a natural massage oil, use Dynasty Sesame Seed Oil, an emollient extracted from sesame seeds that absorbs UV radiation and is a common ingredient in sunscreen lotions. If desired, you can scent sesame seed oil with a few drops of McCormick Mint Extract, McCormick Pure Anise Extract, McCormick Pure Lemon Extract, McCormick Pure Orange Extract, McCormick Pure Peppermint Extract, or McCormick Pure Vanilla Extract (or the pure essential oils listed on the chart on page 5).

■ **Dynasty Sesame Seed Oil, International Collection Sweet Almond Oil, McCormick Ground Cinnamon, McCormick Ground Nutmeg,** and **Mr. Coffee Filters.** To make a sweet massage oil, mix one-quarter cup Dynasty Sesame Seed Oil, two tablespoons International Collection Sweet Almond Oil, one-quarter teaspoon McCormick Ground Cinnamon, and one-quarter teaspoon McCormick Ground Nutmeg. Let stand for three hours, then strain through a Mr. Coffee Filter.

■ **Fleischmann's Margarine.** Massage softened Fleischmann's Margarine over your entire body, let penetrate the skin, then shower clean in warm water. The vegetable oils in the margarine soften skin.

■ **French's Mustard.** Massage a generous amount of French's Mustard into sore muscles and then cover with a washcloth dampened with warm water as a soothing poultice. Wait fifteen minutes, allowing the heat from the mustard to penetrate your body, then rinse clean.

■ Fruit of the Earth Aloe Vera Gel. Massage Fruit of the Earth Aloe Vera Gel into tight muscles to cool, soothe, and tingle the stiffness and aches.

■ Gatorade. To soothe and rejuvenate achy muscles, drink Gatorade, which quickly replenishes the body with carbohydrates. The body converts carbohydrates into glycogen—a fuel for muscles.

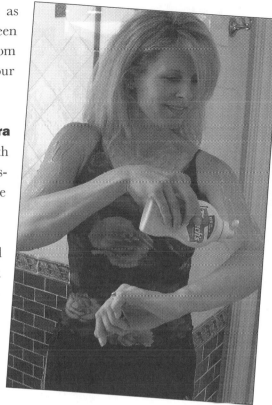

■ Gold's Horseradish and **Star Olive Oil.** Mix one tablespoon Gold's Horseradish in one-half cup Star Olive Oil. Let set for thirty minutes to allow the horseradish to infuse the oil. Massage the spicy oil into sore muscles for instant relief.

■ Grapeola Grape Seed Oil. This all-natural oil extracted from grape seeds makes a wonderful massage oil because it is a non-allergenic emollient and the least greasy oil there is. If desired, you can scent grape seed oil with a few drops of McCormick Mint Extract, McCormick Pure Anise Extract, McCormick Pure Lemon Extract, McCormick Pure Orange Extract, McCormick Pure Peppermint Extract, or McCormick Pure Vanilla Extract (or the pure essential oils listed on the chart on page 5).

■ **Hain Safflower Oil.** For a natural massage oil, use Hain Safflower Oil, an emollient that contains nearly 75 percent linoleic acid. If desired, you can scent safflower oil with a few drops of McCormick Mint Extract, McCormick Pure Anise Extract, McCormick Pure Lemon Extract, McCormick Pure Orange Extract, McCormick Pure Peppermint Extract, or McCormick Pure Vanilla Extract (or the pure essential oils listed on the chart on page 5).

■ **International Collection Sweet Almond Oil.** For a fragrant massage oil, use International Collection Sweet Almond Oil, an emollient that moisturizes the skin. If desired, you can scent almond oil with a few drops of McCormick Mint Extract, McCormick Pure Anise Extract, McCormick Pure Lemon Extract, McCormick Pure Orange Extract, McCormick Pure Peppermint Extract, or McCormick Pure Vanilla Extract (or the pure essential oils listed on the chart on page 5).

■ **Johnson's Baby Powder.** Johnson's Baby Powder works like a massage oil, lubricating the skin to reduce friction without the greasy mess of oil.

■ **Land O Lakes Butter.** Using soft Land O Lakes Butter as a massage oil moisturizes the skin and calms the senses with the familiar aroma of buttered popcorn.

■ **Loriva Extra Sunflower Oil.** Sunflower Oil, extracted from sunflower seeds, makes an excellent massage oil. If desired, you can scent sunflower oil with a few drops of McCormick Mint Extract, McCormick Pure Anise Extract, McCormick Pure Lemon Extract, McCormick Pure Orange Extract, McCormick Pure Peppermint Extract, or McCormick Pure Vanilla Extract (or the pure essential oils listed on the chart on page 5).

■ **Lubriderm.** Using Lubriderm—the moisturizing lotion created in 1946 for dermatologists as a base for their own formulations to treat dry skin—as a massage oil leaves skin soft and moisturized.

■ **McCormick Bay Leaves, Star Olive Oil,** and **Mr. Coffee Filters.** Place three McCormick Bay leaves and four teaspoons Star Olive Oil in a saucepan and warm over low heat. Do not let the oil burn or smoke. Let cool, then strain through a Mr. Coffee Filter. Massage this potent herbal tincture into sore muscles.

■ **McCormick Mint Extract, McCormick Pure Anise Extract, McCormick Pure Lemon Extract, McCormick Pure Orange Extract, McCormick Pure Peppermint Extract,** and/or **McCormick Pure Vanilla Extract.** To enhance your massage with aromatherapy, add a few drops of McCormick Mint Extract, McCormick Pure Anise Extract, McCormick Pure Lemon Extract, McCormick Pure Orange Extract, McCormick Pure Peppermint Extract, or McCormick Pure Vanilla Extract (or any combination of these extracts you please) to whatever carrier oil you intend to use as a massage oil.

■ **Noxzema.** Noxzema, the skin cream originally invented in 1914 by pharmacist Dr. George Bunting in the prescription room of his Baltimore drugstore as a sunburn remedy, doubles as marvelous massage cream. The camphor, menthol, and eucalyptus oil also provide soothing aromatherapy.

■ **Pam Cooking Spray.** It's aerosol massage oil! Simply spray some Pam Cooking Spray on your skin and rub away all that tension and tightness.

■ **Skin-So-Soft.** To alleviate the tightness of sore muscles, use Skin-So-Soft as a fragrant massage oil.

■ **Star Olive Oil.** This restorative emollient with a light fragrance makes a moisturizing massage oil. If desired, you can scent olive oil with a few drops of McCormick Mint Extract, McCormick Pure Anise Extract, McCormick Pure Lemon Extract, McCormick Pure Orange Extract, McCormick Pure Peppermint Extract, or McCormick Pure Vanilla Extract (or the pure essential oils listed on the chart on page 5).

■ **Tabasco Pepper Sauce.** Massage the hot sauce into your back, neck, and sore muscles. The alkaloid capsaicin in Tabasco Pepper Sauce deadens pain when applied topically. Capsaicin enters nerves and temporarily depletes them of the neurotransmitter that sends pain signals to the brain. If you feel any burning, apply some Colgate Toothpaste over the dried Tabasco Pepper Sauce. The glycerin in the toothpaste minimizes the sting and may also boost the capsaicin's analgesic properties. Do not apply Tabasco Pepper Sauce to an open wound.

■ **Uncle Ben's Converted Brand Rice.** Fill a sock with uncooked Uncle Ben's Converted Brand Rice (not too compactly), tie a knot in the end, and heat it in the microwave for four or five minutes. Place the warm sock on your back, neck, forehead, or over your eyes or sore muscles for ten minutes. The reusable heating pad conforms wherever applied.

■ **Wesson Canola Oil.** This fragrant emollient makes an excellent massage oil that moisturizes skin. If desired, you can scent canola oil with a few drops of McCormick Mint Extract, McCormick Pure Anise Extract, McCormick Pure Lemon Extract, McCormick Pure Orange Extract, McCormick Pure Peppermint Extract, or McCormick Pure Vanilla Extract (or the pure essential oils listed on the chart on page 5).

■ **Wilson Tennis Balls.** Put several Wilson Tennis Balls inside a sock, tie a knot at the end, and have a friend roll this over your back. This technique is frequently used by labor coaches to massage the backs of pregnant women in labor.

■ **Ziploc Freezer Bags.** A gallon-size Ziploc Freezer Bag makes an excellent inflatable portable back pillow. Simply seal the bag securely, leaving a half-inch opening at one end of the "zipper." Inflate the bag and quickly seal the remaining half-inch. Place behind the small of your back when sitting in an office chair, driving the car, or riding on long airplane flights. Deflate and flatten for easy storage.

■ **Ziploc Freezer Bags.** Heat soothes muscle, back, and neck pain. Fill a gallon-size Ziploc Freezer Bag with hot water, seal securely, and place on your back, letting the flexible hot water bottle conform to the shape of your body.

■ **Ziploc Freezer Bags.** Applying an ice pack to your back, neck, or sore muscles for ten minutes relieves aches and pains. Fill a Ziploc Freezer Bag with water and freeze it or fill it with ice cubes. Wrap the ice pack in a paper towel before applying. For more ways to make and apply an ice pack, see page 55.

■ **Ziploc Storage Bags.** When applying BenGay or Therapeutic Mineral Ice, wear a Ziploc Storage Bag over each one of your hands to avoid getting the hot gel on your hands.

Immerse Yourself

■ When applied to the skin, diluted essential oils enter the pores and get absorbed into the bloodstream or lymphatic system, where they are believe to help lower blood pressure, stimulate circulation, promote detoxification, and enhance healthy cell renewal.

■ According to the National Institutes of Health, an estimated twenty million Americans receive massage therapy and bodywork each year.

■ One out of every three Americans has tried massage therapy.

■ Massage therapy eases pain, relieves stress, controls cardiovascular and neurological ailments, soothes headaches, speeds recovery from illness, nourishes the skin, increases lymphatic and blood circulation, stimulates the production of endorphins, and eliminates toxins from the body.

■ For a massage at home, lie on a beach towel on the floor and cover it with a cotton bed sheet.

■ Massage oil reduces the friction created by rubbing the skin.

■ The Chinese practiced massage as early as 3000 B.C.E., focusing on specific points along the body's "meridians," channels through which energy travels through the body.

■ In the seventh century C.E., the Japanese developed shiatsu massage (finger pressure or acupressure).

■ The Vedas, the oldest sacred books of Hinduism, written around 1000 B.C.E., contain the Ayurveda, a comprehensive medical system that includes massage for sensual purposes.

■ Ancient Greek physician Hippocrates advised his fellow physicians to learn massage as part of their treatment practices. "Hard rubbing binds," said Hippocrates. "Much rubbing causes parts to waste…and moderate rubbing makes them grow."

■ In Ancient Rome, Julius Caesar used massage therapy to relieve his neuralgia and epileptic seizures.

■ In the early 1850s, Swedish physiologist Peter Henry Ling developed a formal system of massage known as "Swedish massage."

■ The basic strokes in Swedish massage are effleurage (slow, long, rhythmic strokes made with the flattened palm of the hand), kneading (grasping the fatty areas of the body as if kneading bread), petrissage (using the fingers to knead soft tissue in small, circular motions), percussion (giving a rapid succession of gentle karate chops), and friction (rubbing the palms rapidly over the body).

Moisturizing

■ **Alberto VO5 Conditioning Hairdressing.** Rub a dab of Alberto VO5 Conditioning Hairdressing over damp skin to seal in moisture.

■ **Bag Balm.** Moisturize dry hands, feet, or face by rubbing on Bag Balm, the salve created in Vermont to help farmers relieve cracking in cow udders.

■ **Castor Oil.** This natural emollient—first used as a skin softener throughout Mesopotamia and ancient Egypt—doubles as a nourishing moisturizer.

■ **ChapStick.** Rubbing ChapStick into dry skin anywhere on your body (face, hands, elbows, knees, feet) seals in moisture and heals chapping, dry skin.

■ **Cool Whip.** Applying Cool Whip as a skin cream moisturizes the skin thanks to the coconut and palm kernel oils in the dessert topping.

■ **Coppertone.** Rubbing Coppertone sunscreen into your hands moisturizes the skin while simultaneously protecting them from sunburn. The emollients in Coppertone—jojoba oil, palm oil, and aloe—rejuvenate dry skin.

■ **Cortaid.** Every time you finish washing your hands, rub a small dab of this hydrocortisone cream into your hands. Then cover your hands a moisturizing lubricant.

■ **Crisco All-Vegetable Shortening.** After washing your face with warm water or after taking a shower, moisturize your face or your entire body with Crisco All-Vegetable Shortening.

■ **Dannon Yogurt.** Before taking a shower, cover your entire body with Dannon Plain Yogurt (add an optional teaspoon of Star Olive Oil, if desired), wait ten minutes, then rinse clean with warm water. The yogurt moisturizes the skin.

■ **Dynasty Sesame Seed Oil.** For a natural moisturizer, use Dynasty Sesame Seed Oil, an emollient extracted from sesame seeds that absorbs UV radiation and is a common ingredient in sunscreen lotions.

■ **Fleischmann's Margarine.** Massage softened Fleischmann's Margarine over your entire body, let it penetrate the skin, then shower clean in warm water. The vegetable oils in the margarine soften skin.

■ **Fruit of the Earth Aloe Vera Gel.** Rub Fruit of the Earth Aloe Vera Gel into your face and body to soothe and moisturize the skin. This cooling, soothing gel made from Aloe Vera leaves forms a protective barrier that helps skin retain moisture.

■ **Grapeola Grape Seed Oil.** This all-natural oil extracted from grape seeds makes an excellent moisturizer because it is an nonallergenic emollient and the least greasy oil there is.

■ **Hain Safflower Oil.** For a natural moisturizer, rub a few drops of Hain Safflower Oil into your skin.

■ **International Collection Sweet Almond Oil.** For a fragrant moisturizer, use International Collection Sweet Almond Oil, an emollient that rejuvenates the skin.

■ **Johnson's Baby Oil.** Rub a few drops of Johnson's Baby Oil into your body to moisturize dry skin. (Be sure to stay out of the sun. Mineral oil makes your skin more susceptible to sunburn.)

■ **Kingsford's Corn Starch.** Soften your skin by applying Kingsford's Corn Starch as you would baby powder or moisturizer. The corn starch seals in moisture.

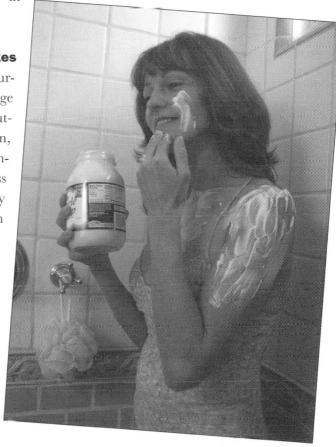

■ **Land O Lakes Butter.** To moisturize skin, massage Land O Lakes Butter into your skin, wait fifteen minutes, remove excess butter with Bounty Paper Towels, then take a hot bath.

■ **Loriva Extra Sunflower Oil.** A few drops of sunflower oil, extracted from sunflower seeds, makes an excellent moisturizer, leaving skin soft and smooth.

■ **McCormick Mint Extract, McCormick Pure Anise Extract, McCormick Pure Lemon Extract, McCormick Pure Orange Extract, McCormick Pure Peppermint Extract**, and/or **McCormick**

Pure Vanilla Extract. To enhance natural oils with aromatherapy, add a few drops of McCormick Mint Extract, McCormick Pure Anise Extract, McCormick Pure Lemon Extract, McCormick Pure Orange Extract, McCormick Pure Peppermint Extract, or McCormick Pure Vanilla Extract (or any combination of these extracts you please) to whatever carrier oil you intend to use as a moisturizer.

■ **McCormick Pure Vanilla Extract** and **Crisco All-Vegetable Shortening.** Mix one-half tablespoon McCormick Pure Vanilla Extract and one tablespoon Crisco All-Vegetable Shortening and massage the mixture into your hands. The vanilla provides aromatherapy, and the shortening moisturizes the skin.

■ **Miracle Whip.** Applying Miracle Whip as a skin cream moisturizes the skin and exfoliates dead skin cells. Let set for a few minutes, then massage with your fingertips.

■ **Noxzema.** Noxzema, the skin cream originally invented in 1914 by pharmacist Dr. George Bunting in the prescription room of his Baltimore drugstore as a sunburn remedy, moisturizes skin.

■ **Pam Cooking Spray.** Spray your body with a very light coat of Pam Cooking Spray and rub into the skin. The oils in the cooking spray moisturize dry skin.

■ **Preparation H.** For dry, chapped skin, apply a dab of Preparation H and rub into your hands and body as a moisturizer.

■ **Quaker Oats, SueBee Honey,** and **ReaLemon.** In a blender, grind two cup Quaker Oats into a fine powder. In a bowl, mix the powdered Quaker Oats with enough SueBee Honey and ReaLemon lemon juice to make a thick paste. Apply the sticky substance to your body, let sit for ten minutes, then rinse with warm water.

The oats absorbs the oils from the skin, the citric acid in the lemon juice disinfects the pores, and the honey is hygroscopic, moisturizing the skin.

■ **ReaLemon** and **Star Olive Oil.** Rejuvenate dry skin by applying ReaLemon lemon juice, rinsing clean, and then rubbing in Star Olive Oil.

■ **Skippy Peanut Butter.** To exfoliate and moisturize dry hands, elbows, and knees, rub the skin with crunchy Skippy Peanut Butter. Let set for ten minutes, then wipe your hands clean with a sheet of Bounty Paper Towel. Rinse clean in warm water. The oils in the peanut butter moisturize skin, the fatty acids soften dry skin, and the nuts exfoliate.

■ **Star Olive Oil.** Warm one-half cup Star Olive Oil in a microwave oven until slightly warm to the touch and massage this restorative emollient into dry skin.

■ **Vaseline Petroleum Jelly.** To moisturize your face, wash your face thoroughly and, while still wet, rub in a small dab of Vaseline Petroleum Jelly. (A dab of Vaseline Petroleum Jelly cleans mascara, eyeliner, lipstick, and rouge from your face, while simultaneously moisturizing the skin.) To moisturize your hands or feet, before going to bed, rub Vaseline Petroleum Jelly into your hands or feet, put on a pair of cotton gloves or socks, and go to sleep. In the morning, your hands or feet will be remarkably soft.

■ **Wesson Canola Oil.** A few drops of this fragrant emollient, rubbed into your body, moisturizes skin.

■ **Wesson Corn Oil** and **Bounty Paper Towels.** Massage Wesson Corn Oil into your skin, wait fifteen minutes, remove the excess oil with a Bounty Paper Towel, and then take a hot bath.

Immerse Yourself

■ To select the proper moisturizer for your skin, test the moisturizer on your skin to determine whether if feels hot or cold. Moisturizer for oily skin should leave your skin feeling cool because it evaporates quickly. Moisturizer for dry skin should leave your skin feeling warm because it remains on the skin surface.

■ The best way to moisturize skin is to drink water, ideally eight glasses daily. Drinking water revitalizes the skin cells—composed of 80 percent water—giving skin its soft and supple look.

■ Moisturizer rehydrates and nourishes the skin and helps the skin cells retain moisture by fortifying the hydrolipidic film on the surface of the skin.

■ Moisturizers do not replenish all the moisture in your skin. They provide some moisture, but moisturizers primarily protect the moisture already in your skin.

■ When moisturizing your face, a dollop of moisturizer the size of a quarter is plenty. Using more moisturizer than that is wasteful.

■ If you have oily skin or acne, avoid moisturizers, which can clog pores, worsening your problem.

■ All commercial moisturizers basically do the same thing.

■ After twenty-five years of age, the natural oil and moisture level of skin decreases, muscle tone declines, and blood circulation weakens, causing skin to dry and wrinkle.

■ Skin holds one-fifth of the body's total water content.

■ Moisturizers fall into two major categories: humectants (oil in water emulsions, better known as lotions) and occlusives (water in oil formulations, better known as creams).

■ Absorbed into the skin, moisturizers plump out fine wrinkles temporarily, creating the false illusion that wrinkles have been eliminated.

Mousse

■ **Budweiser.** Open a can of Budweiser beer and let it sit at room temperature until it goes flat. Pour the beer into a trigger-spray bottle. After a shower, towel dry your hair and then spray your hair lightly with beer before blow-drying, curling, or setting. The odor evaporates quickly, and your hair sets without smelling like beer.

■ **C&H Cane Sugar.** Dissolve one part C&H Cane Sugar with two parts warm water in a trigger-spray bottle and spray your hair with a light coat of the sweet hair spray. The liquid evaporates, setting your hair in place.

■ **Close-Up Classic Red Gel Toothpaste.** Squeeze a dollop of Close-Up Classic Red Gel Toothpaste into your palm, rub your palms together, and then rub the toothpaste spike your hair. The gel holds any hairstyle in place, making your head kissably fresh.

■ **Coca-Cola.** Mix equal parts Coca-Cola and water in a trigger-spray bottle and shake well. After getting out of the shower or bath, towel dry your hair, and then spray a light coat of the diluted Coke over your hair to give your locks a tousled look.

■ **Coppertone.** In a pinch, Coppertone sunscreen doubles as hair gel. Squeeze a dollop of Coppertone into your palm, rub your palms together, and then rub the sunscreen through your hair.

■ **Dickinson's Witch Hazel.** Too much styling gel or other product in your hair? Blot with a cotton ball saturated with Dickinson's Witch Hazel to dissolve the product.

■ **Elmer's Glue-All.** Squeeze a dollop of Elmer's Glue-All in the palm of your hand, rub your hands together, and comb your fingers through your hair to apply the glue evenly to your hair. Comb your hair with a fine-tooth comb to remove the excess glue (wash the glue off the comb under running water). Style your hair to your liking (spike if you wish) and let the glue dry. (Elmer's Glue-All is water soluble and washes out of hair with regular shampoo.)

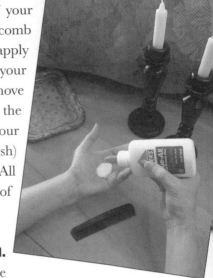

■ **Fruit of the Earth Aloe Vera Gel.** Mousse your hair with Fruit of the Earth Aloe Vera Gel, which doubles as hairstyling gel.

■ **Gillette Foamy.** A small dab of Gillette Foamy combed through your hair will keep it in place. If you use a blow-dryer with shaving cream in your hair, you can make your hair stand up on end.

■ **Jell-O.** Rub a dab of your favorite flavor of ready-made Jell-O through your hair and comb. The gelatin works just like mousse. Or use one teaspoon Jell-O powder dissolved in one cup water.

■ **Johnson's Baby Oil.** After brushing your hair, rub a dab of Johnson's Baby Oil between your palms and then run your hands through your hair for an amazing shine.

■ **Lubriderm.** Rub a dollop of unscented Lubriderm between your palms and then run your fingers through soft hair to firm it up.

■ **Phillips' Milk of Magnesia.** Mix two tablespoons Phillips' Milk of Magnesia in one cup water in a trigger-spray bottle. Spray the mixture in your hair, comb well to spread the setting solution equally, style your hair, and let dry.

■ **Sprite.** Pour a can of Sprite into a trigger-spray bottle and lightly mist the ends of curly or wavy hair to hold it in place.

■ **Star Olive Oil.** After brushing your hair, rub a dab of Star Olive Oil between your palms and then run your hands through your hair for an amazing shine.

■ **Vaseline Petroleum Jelly.** After brushing your hair, rub a dab of Vaseline Petroleum Jelly between your palms and then run your hands through your hair to hold it in place with a remarkable shine.

Immerse Yourself

■ Man-made combs dating back to 4000 B.C.E. have been found in Egyptian tombs.

■ The earliest known comb is believed to be the dried backbone of a large fish.

■ In 1920, two companies in Racine, Wisconsin—the Racine Universal Motor Company and Hamilton Beach—essentially combined the vacuum cleaner with the blender to create the hand-held hair dryer. The Racine Universal Motor Company introduced the "Race"; Hamilton Beach launched the "Cyclone."

■ In 1951, Sears, Roebuck and Co. introduced a portable hand-held dryer that attached to a pink plastic cap that fit over the woman's hair.

■ In 1968, Leandro P. Rizzuto, founder of Continental Hair Products in New York City, developed the hot comb, and three years later, he introduced the first hand-held pistol-grip blow-dryer to the United States.

Mud Packs & Body Wraps

■ **BenGay** and **Saran Wrap.** Apply BenGay to any sore spot, then wrap the area with Saran Wrap. The plastic wrap increases the heat of the liniment. Be careful not to burn the skin.

■ **Carnation NonFat Dry Milk.** Mix one cup Carnation NonFat Dry Milk with enough water to make a thick paste. Apply the milky paste to your body, let dry, then wash off. The milk moisturizes and nourishes the skin, giving you a radiant glow.

■ **Carnation NonFat Dry Milk, Bigelow Plantation Mint Classic Tea Bags, McCormick Rosemary Leaves, McCormick Pure Peppermint Extract,** and **Saran Wrap.** To make an excellent foot wrap, mix three ounces Carnation NonFat Dry Milk and eight ounces warm water in a wide bowl. Add the contents of one Bigelow Plantation Mint Classic Tea Bag, one teaspoon McCormick Rosemary Leaves, and one teaspoon McCormick Pure Peppermint Extract. Using a washcloth, apply the solution to your feet, wrap in Saran Wrap, wait five minutes, and rinse clean.

■ **Carnation NonFat Dry Milk, SueBee Honey,** and **Dynasty Sesame Seed Oil.** Mix four tablespoons Carnation NonFat Dry Milk powder with enough hot water to make a thin paste, the consistency of mustard. Mix three tablespoons SueBee Honey and one tablespoon Dynasty Sesame Seed Oil in a bowl and warm in a microwave oven. Apply the honey and sesame seed oil mixture to your body and lie down on a towel or cotton sheet for ten minutes. Using a washcloth saturated with the warm milk paste, wipe the honey and oil mixture from your skin. Lie on the towel or cotton sheet for another ten minutes, then rinse clean in a warm shower.

■ **Cool Whip.** Cover your body with Cool Whip. Let set twenty minutes, then wash clean with warm water followed by cold water. The coconut and palm kernel oils moisturize the skin.

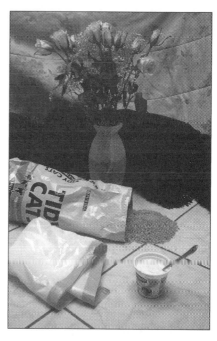

■ **Dannon Yogurt, Tidy Cats,** and **Glad Trash Bags.** Cut open one or two large Glad Trash Bags to create a large rectangle of plastic. Mix one cup Dannon Plain Yogurt with one cup Tidy Cats Regular Clay to make a thick, muddy paste. Using a paintbrush, gravy brush, or spatula, spread the mud evenly over your body to create an all-body mask, starting with your feet and working your way up to your face, gently massaging the mixture into your skin. Wrap yourself in the Glad Trash Bags and wait a half hour for the mud to dry. Shower clean with warm water, followed by a quick rinse with cold water. Pat dry with a towel and moisturize well. The clay from the cat box filler detoxifies your skin by absorbing dirt and oil from the pores, while the yogurt soothes your skin.

■ **Dole Crushed Pineapple, Thai Kitchen Coconut Milk,** and **Glad Trash Bags.** Cut open one or two large Glad Trash Bags to create a large rectangle of plastic and spread them on the bottom of a bathtub. In a blender, mix three cups Dole Crushed Pineapple and one cup Thai Kitchen Coconut Milk. Lying in the bathtub on top of the Glad Trash Bags, rub the mixture all over your skin, and then wrap yourself in the plastic. Wait twenty minutes, then unwrap the plastic wrap and shower clean with cool water.

■ **French's Mustard** and **Glad Trash Bags.** Cut open one or two large Glad Trash Bags to create a large rectangle of plastic. Starting with your feet and working your way up to your face, rub French's Mustard all over your body and then wrap your legs, arms, and torso in the plastic trash bags. Wait twenty minutes, then shower clean with warm water, followed by a quick rinse with cold water. Mustard both stimulates and soothes the skin by causing a rise in temperature, and being wrapped in plastic also raises the body's temperature, causing profuse perspiration that eliminates impurities and toxins.

■ **Fruit of the Earth Aloe Vera Gel, SueBee Honey,** and **Kingsford's Corn Starch.** Mix equal parts Fruit of the Earth Aloe Vera Gel and SueBee Honey, blend thoroughly, then add enough Kingsford's Corn Starch to bring the consistency of the mixture to the thickness of a cream. Spread the mixture over your body, let dry thoroughly, then rub off with a wet washcloth to gently exfoliate the skin.

■ **Heinz Apple Cider Vinegar.** Pour one cup Heinz Apple Cider Vinegar in one gallon warm water. Soak a towel in the solution and wrap it around the area of the body that ails you. The warm vinegar helps heat up the body and improve circulation.

■ **Hershey's Cocoa** and **SueBee Honey.** Mix three-quarters cup Hershey's Cocoa powder and one-quarter cup SueBee Honey in a microwave-safe bowl. Warm the sticky mixture in a microwave oven. Let the paste cool to the touch and then apply all over your body. Wait twenty minutes, then shower clean.

■ **Libby's Pumpkin.** To get your skin silky soft, cover your body with a thin coat of pumpkin, let dry, and then rinse clean. Pumpkin, loaded with vitamin A and fruit acid enzymes, moisturizes and conditions the skin.

■ **Maxwell House Coffee** and **Glad Trash Bags.** Cut open one or two large Glad Trash Bags to create a large rectangle of plastic. To reduce cellulite, take freshly used Maxwell House Coffee grounds and rub the warm grounds all over your body from the neck down (or wherever cellulite is giving your trouble). Wrap yourself up in the plastic trash bags and use a rolling pin to roll over the plastic wrap. Rinse clean.

■ **Miracle Whip.** Using a paintbrush or spatula, apply Miracle Whip as an all-body mask. Miracle Whip cleanses the skin and tightens the pores. Leave it on for twenty minutes and then wash off with warm water, followed by cold water.

■ **Pepto-Bismol** and **Reynolds Wrap.** Using a paintbrush, cover your body with Pepto-Bismol and then wrap your legs, arms, and torso in Reynolds Wrap. Sit twenty minutes, then rinse clean with warm water, followed by cool water. Pepto-Bismol absorbs oils from the skin and tightens the pores, leaving your skin looking smoother and feeling softer.

■ **Phillips' Milk of Magnesia.** Apply Phillips' Milk of Magnesia as a full-body mask, let dry for thirty minutes, then rinse off with warm water, followed by cool water. The milk of magnesia absorbs the oils from your skin, while simultaneously cooling the skin.

■ **Quaker Oats, SueBee Honey,** and **ReaLemon.** In a blender, grind two cup Quaker Oats into a fine powder. In a bowl, mix the powdered Quaker Oats with enough SueBee Honey and ReaLemon lemon juice to make a thick paste. Apply the sticky substance to your face, let sit for ten minutes, then rinse with warm water. The oats absorbs the oils from the skin, the citric acid in the lemon juice disinfects the pores, and the honey is hygroscopic, moisturizing the skin.

■ **Saran Wrap.** If wrapping yourself in Glad Trash Bags is too cumbersome, wrap yourself in Saran Wrap.

■ **SueBee Honey, Carnation Evaporated Milk, Heinz Apple Cider Vinegar,** and **Gold Medal Flour.** Mix six tablespoons SueBee Honey, one cup Carnation Evaporated Milk, and one-third cup Heinz Apple Cider Vinegar in a bowl. Then add enough Gold Medal Flour to make a very thick paste. Apply as an all-body mask and let dry. Rinse with warm water, followed by cold water. The honey disinfects the skin and seals in moisture, the milk moisturizes, and the vinegar tightens the pores.

■ **Tidy Cats, Mott's Apple Juice, ReaLemon, International Collection Sweet Almond Oil, SueBee Honey,** and **Reynolds Wrap.** Mix six ounces Tidy Cats Regular Clay, seven fluid ounces Mott's Apple Juice, and one tablespoon ReaLemon lemon juice to form a smooth paste. Add two tablespoons International Collection Sweet Almond Oil, one tablespoon SueBee Honey, and six drops sandalwood essential oil. Using a paintbrush or spatula, spread the mud evenly over your body, starting with your feet and working your way up to your face, gently massaging the mixture into your skin. Wrap yourself in Reynolds Wrap and wait a half hour for the mud to dry. Shower clean with warm water, followed by a rinse with cold water. Pat dry with a towel and moisturize well. The clay from the cat box filler detoxifies your skin by absorbing dirt and oil from the pores, the apple juice soothes the skin, the lemon juice is a natural antiseptic, and the honey disinfects the skin and seals in moisture.

■ **Wesson Corn Oil, Ocean Spray Grapefruit Juice, McCormick Ground Thyme,** and **Glad Trash Bags.** Cut open one or two large Glad Trash Bags to create a large rectangle of plastic. To fight cellulite, mix one cup Wesson Corn Oil, one-half cup Ocean Spray Grapefruit Juice, and two teaspoons McCormick Ground Thyme in a bowl. Massage the mixture into your thighs and buttocks, cover with the Glad Trash Bags, and wait ten minutes. Rinse clean with warm water.

Immerse Yourself

■ Mud therapy is also known as fangotherapy, from the Italian word *fango*, meaning mud.

■ No one knows exactly how mud therapy works. By coating the human body in warm mud and then wrapping it in foil, the mud dries, absorbing excess oils, tightening the pores, softening the skin, and raising the body temperature, causing profuse sweating, which expels toxins from the body.

■ Mud therapy relieves and relaxes muscles and aids in the healing of stressed joints.

■ Mud used in spa treatments is usually a clay base to which natural ingredients like algae, kelp, herbs, minerals, peat moss, paraffin, or essential oils have been added.

■ The phrase "Your name is Mudd" refers to Samuel Mudd, the doctor who set the broken leg of President Abraham Lincoln's assassin, John Wilkes Booth.

■ Muddy Waters, the kingpin of the Chicago blues scene best known for his hit songs "Rollin' Stone," "(I'm Your) Hoochie Coochie Man," and "I'm Ready," initially earned a living driving a truck for a venetian-blind manufacturer in Mississippi. One of his albums is entitled "Electric Mud."

■ In 1985, singer and actress Bette Midler released an album entitled "Mud Will Be Flung Tonight."

Rubs & Scrubs

■ **Albers Corn Meal.** Make a paste from Albers Corn Meal and water, apply to skin, massage well, wait ten minutes, then wash clean with warm water. The corn meal cleanses the skin.

■ **Arm & Hammer Baking Soda.** Mix one-half cup Arm & Hammer Baking Soda with water to form a paste. Massage the mixture over your skin, and then rinse clean with warm water, followed by cool water. Pat dry with a towel. The baking soda cleanses the pores and exfoliates dead skin.

■ **Baker's Angel Flake Coconut, McCormick Ground Turmeric, Gerber Carrots,** and **Knox Gelatin.** Mix one-half cup Baker's Angel Flake Coconut with one-quarter teaspoon McCormick Ground Turmeric. Take a shower, and before toweling yourself dry, rub the coconut and turmeric mixture over your damp skin. Wait five minutes, then wipe off with a warm cloth. Mix eight ounces Gerber carrots with two tablespoons Knox Gelatin powder and apply the mixture to your skin. Wait five minutes, then rinse clean and towel dry.

■ **C&H Brown Sugar** and **McCormick Pure Vanilla Extract.** Place one teaspoon C&H Brown Sugar in your palm, cover with McCormick Pure Vanilla Extract, and buff your skin. The sugar granules exfoliate dry skin and the vanilla extract provides a delicious scent. Rinse clean and pat dry with a towel.

■ **C&H Cane Sugar** and **Wesson Vegetable Oil.** Mix one tablespoon C&H Cane Sugar and one tablespoon Wesson Vegetable

Oil in the cupped palm of your hand, rub the coarse goo into your hands, elbows, and knees to exfoliate dead skin cells, and then rinse clean with cold water. The gritty granules exfoliate dead cells while the vegetable oil moisturizes the skin.

■ **Carnation NonFat Dry Milk.** Mix one-half cup Carnation NonFat Dry Milk with enough water to make a thick paste. Massage the milky paste all over your body and face and then rinse clean. The lactic acids remove grime and exfoliate dead skin, and the proteins in the milk leave the skin feeling silky smooth.

■ **Cheerios.** Using a blender, grind one cup Cheerios into a fine powder. Rub the pulverized oats over your body to exfoliate the dry skin. Wash with cool water, dry well, then apply moisturizer.

■ **Country Time Lemonade.** Mix three tablespoons Country Time Lemonade powdered drink with enough water to make a thick paste. Massage the lemony paste over your skin (avoiding your eyes), wait five minutes, then rinse clean. The gritty paste and citric acid help exfoliate dead skin, leaving your skin smooth and soft. (Using citric acid on your skin makes you more prone to sunburn, so be sure to use sunscreen afterward.)

■ **Dannon Yogurt.** In a blender, mix one cup Dannon Plain Yogurt with three sprigs fresh peppermint and two sprigs fresh spearmint in a blender for three seconds. Refrigerate the mixture for twenty-four hours to allow the mint to infuse the yogurt. Stir one cup rice flour into the mixture and add one drop peppermint essential oil. Mix well. Rub the creamy solution all over your body by hand or with a loofah. Rinse clean in the shower.

■ **Diamond Chopped Walnuts, Star Olive Oil,** and **SueBee Honey.** Using a mortar and pestle, grind one-half cup Diamond Chopped Walnuts into a fine powder. Add two tablespoons Star

Olive Oil and one tablespoon SueBee Honey. Rub the mixture over your hands and lower arms for several minutes. Rinse clean.

■ **Dole Pineapple Slices.** While taking a shower, rub Dole Pineapple Slices over your skin. Cleanse with a mild soap and rinse clean. The enzymes in the pineapple exfoliate dead skin cells.

■ **Epsom Salt.** To cleanse your skin and exfoliate dead cells, massage handfuls Epsom Salt over your wet skin, staring with your feet and working your way up toward your face. Top off this treatment by pouring two cups of Epsom Salt into a bath of warm water and soaking in the soothing solution for fifteen to twenty minutes. The magnesium sulfate will soften your skin and soothe any sore muscles you may have.

■ **Hodgson Mill Wheat Germ.** Use Hodgson Mill Wheat Germ as a gentle scrub for dry or normal skin.

■ **International Collection Sweet Almond Oil, Dannon Yogurt, Morton Salt,** and **Albers Corn Meal.** To exfoliate dead skin cells from callused elbows and knees, mix three tablespoons International Collection Sweet Almond Oil, two tablespoons Dannon Plain Yogurt, two tablespoons Morton Salt, and two tablespoons Albers Corn Meal in a bowl. In the shower, rub this scrub over your elbows and knees with a washcloth or vegetable brush. Rinse clean and pat dry with a towel.

■ **L'eggs Sheer Energy Panty Hose.** With a pair of scissors, cut off one leg of a pair of clean, used L'eggs Sheer Energy Panty Hose, hold one end of the stocking in each hand, and seesaw it across your back in the bathtub or shower to increase circulation and exfoliate the skin.

■ **L'eggs Sheer Energy Panty Hose.** Using a pair of scissors, cut off the foot from a clean, used pair of L'eggs Sheer Energy Panty Hose and put it over your hairbrush. Before using a rub or scrub or before taking a shower or bath, run the nylon-covered brush over your skin to increase circulation and exfoliate the skin.

■ **Libby's Pumpkin, McCormick Ground Nutmeg, C&H Cane Sugar,** and **SueBee Honey.** Refrigerate a can of Libby's Pumpkin overnight, mix one cup with one teaspoon McCormick Ground Nutmeg, and massage all over dry skin. Pumpkin, loaded with vitamin A and fruit acid enzymes, exfoliates dead skin. Rinse clean, then apply a mixture of equal parts C&H Cane Sugar and SueBee Honey. Wait five minutes, then rinse clean and pat dry with a towel.

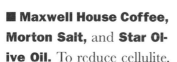

■ **Maxwell House Coffee, Morton Salt,** and **Star Olive Oil.** To reduce cellulite, mix one cup warm, used Maxwell House Coffee grounds, one-half cup Morton Salt, and four tablespoons Star Olive Oil. Rub the warm mixture wherever cellulite is giving your trouble and massage in a circular motion with your hands or using a loofah. Rinse clean and pat dry with a towel.

■ **Miracle Whip.** Exfoliate dead skin by rubbing a dab of Miracle Whip into your feet, knees, elbows, or face. Let set for a few minute, then massage with your fingertips.

■ **Morton Rock Salt, Star Olive Oil,** and **ReaLemon.** For dry skin, mix four tablespoons Morton Rock Salt, one-half cup Star Olive Oil, and two teaspoons ReaLemon lemon juice. Rub the mixture over dry skin on the body (not the face) and rinse clean in a warm shower, using a washcloth.

■ **Morton Salt** and **Johnson's Baby Oil.** Mix equal parts Morton Salt and Johnson's Baby Oil to make an abrasive, moisturizing scrub to exfoliate dry skin. (If you don't have any baby oil, simply mix one part Morton Salt to two parts water.)

■ **Ocean Spray Grapefruit Juice** and **C&H Cane Sugar.** Add enough Ocean Spray Grapefruit Juice to one cup C&H Cane Sugar to make a thick paste. Use this mixture as a scrub to exfoliate dry skin (but not over recently shaved skin or sensitive areas). The citric acid in the grapefruit juice and the coarse sugar granules efficiently exfoliate the skin.

■ **Quaker Oats** and **Albers Corn Meal.** Mix equal parts Quaker Oats and Albers Corn Meal with enough hot water to make a paste. Let cool to a warm temperature and apply the mixture to your skin. Wait ten minutes and then rinse clean with warm water. Pat dry with a towel.

■ **Quaker Oats, C&H Brown Sugar, Fruit of the Earth Aloe Vera Gel,** and **ReaLemon.** Grind up six teaspoons Quaker Oats in a coffee grinder or blender and then mix in a bowl with six teaspoons C&H Brown Sugar, six tablespoons Fruit of the Earth Aloe Vera Gel, and one teaspoon ReaLemon lemon juice to create a smooth paste. Take a shower and before toweling dry, gently massage the mixture onto damp skin. Rinse off with warm water.

■ **Quaker Oats** and **Carnation Evaporated Milk.** Blend four teaspoons Quaker Oats into a fine powder and then mix the powder with two teaspoons Carnation Evaporated Milk. Apply to your skin, rub lightly, then rinse clean.

■ **Quaker Oats** and **International Collection Sweet Almond Oil.** Blend four teaspoons Quaker Oats into a fine powder and then mix the powder with two tablespoons International Collection Sweet Almond oil. Apply to your skin, rub lightly, then rinse clean.

■ **Quaker Oats** and **L'eggs Sheer Energy Panty Hose.** Using a blender, grind one cup Quaker Oats into a fine powder. Cut off the foot from a clean, used pair of L'eggs Sheer Energy Panty Hose, fill with the powdered oats, and tie a knot in the nylon. Tie the oatmeal sachet to the spigot, letting it dangle in the flow of water as the tub fills with warm water. Soak for thirty minutes in this inexpensive and soothing oatmeal bath, then rub the oatmeal sachet over your body to exfoliate and moisturize the skin.

■ **Quaker Oats, Quaker Oat Bran Hot Cereal,** and **Morton Rock Salt.** Mix eight tablespoons Quaker Oats, eight tablespoons Quaker Oat Bran Hot Cereal (dry), and two teaspoons Morton Rock Salt. Add two teaspoons milk and mix to make a thick paste. Rub the paste into the skin with your hands or a body brush. Rinse clean and pat dry with a towel.

■ **R. W. Knudsen Black Cherry Juice** and **Morton Salt.** Mix equal parts R. W. Knudsen Black Cherry Juice and Morton Salt, massage over damp skin, rinse clean, and moisturize. The malic acid in the cherry juice exfoliates dead skin cells and accelerates cell renewal.

■ **ReaLemon** and **Carnation NonFat Dry Milk.** Mix six teaspoons ReaLemon lemon juice and one cup Carnation NonFat Dry Milk to form a paste. Rub into knees, feet, and elbows. Wait fifteen minutes and then scrub off with a washcloth to exfoliate the skin. The citric acid in the lemon juice and the lactic acid in the powdered milk exfoliate dead skin cells.

■ **Scotch-Brite Heavy Duty Scrub Sponge.** Use the coarse side of a Scotch-Brite Heavy Duty Scrub Sponge to gently rub away dead skin.

■ **Scotch Packaging Tape.** Wrap a strip of Scotch Packaging Tape around your hand, adhesive side out, and pat your dry skin. The adhesive will exfoliate the skin.

■ **Skippy Peanut Butter.** To exfoliate and moisturize dry hands, elbows, and knees, rub the skin with crunchy Skippy Peanut Butter. Let set for ten minutes, then wipe your hands clean with a sheet of Bounty Paper Towel. Rinse clean in warm water. The oils in the peanut butter moisturize skin, the fatty acids soften dry skin, and the nuts exfoliate.

■ **Star Olive Oil** and **Morton Salt.** Mix equal parts Star Olive Oil and Morton Salt. Rub the mixture all over your body and then rinse clean in the shower. Pat dry with a soft towel.

Immerse Yourself

■ Exfoliation, using a gentle abrasive on the skin, removes dead cells from the surface of the skin, unblocking pores and enabling them to better absorb creams and oils.

■ Over-scrubbing, over-rubbing, and over-cleansing you skin can cause irritations and wrinkling. Tread lightly.

■ Brushing your body with an exfoliating bath brush (before bathing or showering) removes dead skin cells and boosts circulation, giving your skin a healthy glow.

Shampoos

■ **Aqua Net Hair Spray.** If you don't have time to shampoo your hair, spray it with Aqua Net Hair Spray, then run your fingers through your hair. The alcohol dissolves the oil in your hair.

■ **Arm & Hammer Baking Soda.** Washing your hair once a week with one tablespoon Arm & Hammer Baking mixed with your regular shampoo removes conditioner and styling gel buildup from your hair. Rinse thoroughly, then condition and style as usual.

■ **Arm & Hammer Baking Soda.** To remove chlorine from hair, make a paste from Arm & Hammer Baking Soda and water, apply to hair, and let set for twenty minutes. Rinse clean.

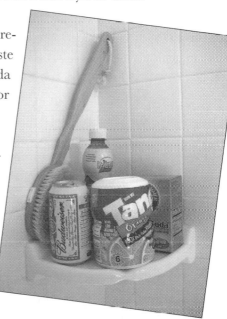

■ **Bayer Aspirin.** Unless you are allergic to aspirin, drop two Bayer Aspirin tablets into your regular shampoo to absorb excess product from the shampoo, enabling the shampoo to clean your hair more effectively.

■ **Budweiser.** Open a can of Budweiser beer and let it sit at room temperature until it goes flat. Shampoo oily hair with the king of beer and rinse thoroughly. Beer absorbs the oils from your hair, but shampooing your hair too often with beer may dry out your scalp, causing dandruff.

■ **Comet.** To cleanse styling gel and hair spray buildup from hair, dissolve one tablespoon Comet (without bleach) in two cups water, pour the solution through your hair (being certain not to get any in your eyes), and let set for three minutes. Shampoo and condition as usual.

■ **Country Time Lemonade.** Pour one tablespoon Country Time Lemonade powdered mix into the palm of your hand, add enough water to make a paste, and use it to shampoo your hair. The citric acid in Country Time Lemonade cuts through sebum oil in hair and leaves your hair smelling lemon fresh.

■ **Dawn Dishwashing Liquid.** Use a few drops of Dawn Dishwashing Liquid as shampoo to cut through grease and grime in hair. The detergent in Dawn thoroughly cleanses hair, stripping styling gel and hair spray buildup from hair.

■ **Dickinson's Witch Hazel.** To remove excess oil from your hair, use a cotton ball to apply Dickinson's Witch Hazel to the roots, then comb through your hair.

■ **Dr. Bronner's Peppermint Soap.** Wet your hair in the shower and use a couple of drops of Dr. Bronner's Peppermint Soap to shampoo your hair. The all-natural ingredients cleanse hair thoroughly, and the peppermint oil leaves your scalp feeling refreshed and invigorated.

■ **Epsom Salt.** For oily hair, mix six tablespoons Epsom Salt in one cup shampoo and use one tablespoon of this mixture to shampoo oily hair. Massage in well, then rinse with cool water. The Epsom Salt absorbs the oil from hair.

■ **Heinz Apple Cider Vinegar.** To rinse styling gel and hair spray buildup from your hair and simultaneously restore natural acids to your mantle, add one tablespoon Heinz Apple Cider Vinegar to a twelve ounce bottle of shampoo, shake well, and use the solution to shampoo your hair. The vinegar also thickens the shampoo (so you use less product, saving money).

■ **Listerine.** For oily hair, after shampooing, use a cotton ball to apply Listerine to your scalp. The antiseptic mouthwash is also an astringent, which slows down oil secretions.

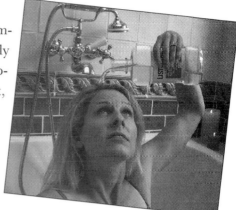

■ **Knox Gelatin.** To thicken your hair, add one packet Knox Gelatin to one-quarter cup shampoo, and wash your hair with the solution.

■ **Mott's Apple Juice** and **Heinz White Vinegar.** For oily hair, mix one cup Mott's Apple Juice and one tablespoon Heinz White Vinegar. After shampooing your hair, pour the mixture through your hair, comb thoroughly, wait fifteen minutes, then shampoo lightly and rinse clean. The pectin in the apple juice, enhanced by the vinegar, absorbs excess oil.

■ **Ocean Spray Grapefruit Juice.** Add one-half cup Ocean Spray Grapefruit Juice to a bottle of shampoo. The acids in the grapefruit juice balance the pH of your hair.

■ **Ocean Spray Grapefruit Juice.** Mix one-half cup Ocean Spray Grapefruit Juice and two cups water in a trigger-spray bottle. After shampooing, spray a fine mist of the solution over your hair. The acids in the grapefruit juice eliminate any remaining buildup of hair products.

■ **ReaLemon.** For oily hair, mix equal parts ReaLemon lemon juice and water. After using your regular shampoo, rinse your hair with the lemon solution.

■ **Smirnoff Vodka.** To cleanse the scalp, remove toxins from hair, stimulate the growth of healthy hair, and leave hair with a great shine, add one jigger Smirnoff Vodka to a twelve-ounce bottle of regular shampoo.

■ **Tang.** Pour one tablespoon Tang drink mix into the palm of your hand, add enough water to make a paste, and use it to shampoo your hair. The citric acid in Tang cuts through sebum oil in hair, and if left in your hair for five minutes, the brightly-colored drink mix adds stylish orange highlights.

■ **Woolite.** To gently strip hair spray and styling gel buildup and simultaneously soften your hair, wash your hair with a capful of Woolite.

DRY SHAMPOO

■ **Arm & Hammer Baking Soda.**
Give yourself a dry shampoo by sprinkling Arm & Hammer Baking Soda in your hair. Work the baking soda into your hair with your fingertips, wait ten minutes, then brush the powder from your hair. The baking soda absorbs sebum oil from hair.

■ **Gold Medal Flour.** When America pioneers crossed the country in covered wagons, the women used handfuls of flour in their hair as a dry shampoo to absorb the oils from their hair. To do the same, simply sprinkle Gold Medal Flour in your hair, work it in with your fingertips, and brush it out.

■ **Huggies Baby Wipes.** If your hair suddenly feels really greasy, use Huggies Baby Wipes to blot excess oil from your roots.

■ **Johnson's Baby Powder.** If you're sick in bed and can't take a shower, give your hair a dry shampoo by working Johnson's Baby Powder into your hair, then brush out.

■ **L'eggs Sheer Energy Panty Hose.** Using a pair of scissors, cut off the foot from a clean, used pair of L'eggs Sheer Energy Panty Hose and put it over your hairbrush. Run the nylon-covered brush through your hair to remove the dirt and oils.

■ **Kingsford's Corn Starch.** Working Kingsford's Corn Starch into your oily hair with your fingertips, waiting five minutes, and then brushing it out absorbs the oils from your hair, giving you a dry shampoo.

■ **Quaker Oats.** Pour dry Quaker Oats into your hair, work the oats into your hair through with your fingertips, and then brush it out. Oats absorb the sebum oil from your hair.

Immerse Yourself

■ The average hair grows roughly one-half inch per month, and the average person loses between fifty and 150 hairs each day.
■ Always shampoo your hair after swimming in a pool, ocean, or salt water lake. Chlorine and salt water damage hair.
■ Inexpensive shampoos tend to clean hair and scalp more effectively than more costly shampoos.

■ Washing your hair with a mild shampoo (that does not strip the acid mantle of the hair)—and then putting moisture back in the hair with a conditioner—keeps hair clean and healthy.

■ The instructions on most commercial shampoo bottles tell us to rinse, lather, and repeat. Shampooing your hair twice usually accomplishes nothing but using twice as much shampoo.

■ Blow-drying, coloring, and changes in your hormones (caused by stress or other factors) can increase pH levels in your hair, reducing the natural shine of your hair. Switching to a shampoo with a lower pH factor can help balance the pH levels in your hair, returning the natural shine.

■ Contrary to popular belief, shampoo alone cannot increase the overall health of the hair.

■ Shampoo merely cleanses excessive sebum (natural oil), body sweat, and environmental impurities from the hair. Stripping the hair of sebum on a daily basis leaves hair more than three inches long exposed to potential damage from the sun, blow-dryers, hair coloring, and permanent waving. Conditioners replace protective oils. To avoid unnecessarily stripping your hair of all sebum, massage shampoo into the first three inches of hair closest to your scalp; when your rinse the shampoo from your hair, the runoff will lightly cleanse the remaining hair.

■ Hair brushes made from animal bristles are porous, which means they help absorb sebum oil from your scalp and distribute it through your hair, giving your hair a consistent shine.

■ Synthetic hair brushes, typically made from nylon, effectively untangle thick hair that tends to get tangles and knots.

■ Paddle brushes help smoothen and dry long hair.

■ Since hair is made from the protein keratin, maintaining healthy hair with a good shine can be achieved by eating a well-balanced diet that includes protein. Massaging the scalp while you shampoo and condition your hair stimulates circulation, bringing protein-rich blood to feed the germinating roots of your hair.

Shaving

■ **Absorbine Jr.** Avoid redness and irritation in the bikini area from shaving by applying Absorbine Jr. to the skin immediately afterward. The Absorbine Jr. stings briefly, but it does prevent itching and red bumps.

■ **Alberto VO5 Conditioning Hairdressing.** Soothe your legs after shaving by rubbing a dollop of Alberto VO5 Conditioning Hairdressing into your skin. The five vital organic ingredients in the hairdressing make your legs feel as smooth as a baby's bottom.

■ **Arm & Hammer Baking Soda.** Minimize razor burn by mixing one tablespoon Arm & Hammer Baking Soda in one cup water and applying the solution to the skin as a protective aftershave lotion.

■ **Cheez Whiz.** All out of shaving cream? Don't panic. Just slather on Cheez Whiz. The oils in the Cheez Whiz lubricate the skin for a close shave and a unique scent.

■ **Clairol Herbal Essences Conditioner.** Instead of using shaving cream on your legs, use Clairol Herbal Essences Conditioner. The lavish emollients in conditioner moisturize the skin, preventing rashes and bumps.

■ **Clean Shower.** Spraying your safety razor blades with Clean Shower after each use triples the life of the razor.

■ **Close-Up Classic Red Gel Toothpaste.** For sensitive skin, use Close-Up Classic Red Gel Toothpaste as a nonallergenic shaving cream, giving a close, smooth shave that leaves the skin feeling slightly anesthetized.

■ **Cool Whip.** Apply Cool Whip to wet skin as shaving cream. The coconut and palm kernel oils in Cool Whip moisturize the skin for a close shave, leaving your skin feeling soft and smooth.

■ **Dr. Bronner's Peppermint Soap.** Fill a sink with water, add two squirts of Dr. Bronner's Peppermint Soap, slather your legs with the soapy water, and shave. The natural oils in the soap moisturize the skin for a close shave.

■ **Heinz White Vinegar.** After shaving, apply Heinz White Vinegar as an aftershave lotion. The vinegar evaporates within an hour and the odor dissipates quickly.

■ **Johnson's Baby Oil.** Rub a few drops of Johnson's Baby Oil into your skin before shaving to raise hair stubs for a clean shave, lubricate the razor, moisturize sensitive skin, and prolong the life of your safety razor blade.

■ **Johnson's Baby Powder.** To prevent friction burns when shaving your legs with an electric razor, dust your legs lightly with Johnson's Baby Powder before shaving.

■ **Land O Lakes Butter.** In a pinch, you can slather Land O Lakes Butter on wet skin for a silky, moisturizing shave.

■ **Lipton Tea Bags.** Got razor burn? Dampen a Lipton Tea bag and place it over the irritated skin. The tannic acid in the tea soothes the redness.

■ **Listerine.** Rinsing your safety razor blade after each use with Listerine sterilizes it and prolongs the life of the razor.

■ **Lubriderm.** If you run out of shaving cream, slather on Lubriderm, which provides a smooth shave and leaves your skin feeling smooth and moisturized.

■ **Miracle Whip.** To avoid razor burn in your bikini area, shave with Miracle Whip, which hydrates the skin and also doubles as shaving cream on your legs.

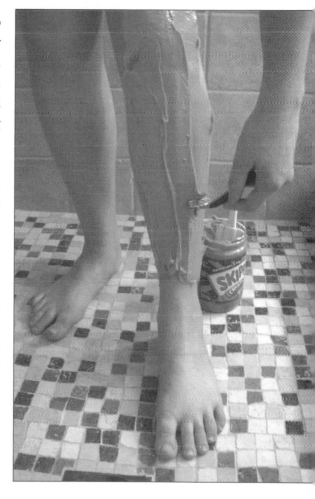

■ **Noxzema.** In a pinch, slather on Noxzema to lubricate the skin for a close shave.

■ **Oral-B Toothbrush.** To clean the stubble from your safety razor, simply brush the blades with a clean, used Oral-B Toothbrush.

■ **Pam Cooking Spray.** Simply spray your legs with this aerosol vegetable oil to lubricate the skin for a smooth shave that leaves the skin luxuriously moisturized.

■ **Reddi-wip.** Spray Reddi-wip whipped cream on your wet skin, rub it in, and shave. The lactic acid in the whipped cream leaves your skin feeling smooth and silky.

■ **Skippy Peanut Butter.** While on a camping trip, former U.S. Senator Barry Goldwater discovered that he could shave with peanut butter. If you're in a pinch, simply slather Skippy Peanut Butter on your legs and shave away. The oils in the peanut butter lubricate the skin for a smooth shave. Just be sure you use the creamy, not the chunky.

■ **Smirnoff Vodka.** After shaving, fill a cup with Smirnoff Vodka and soak your safety razor blade in the alcohol to prolong the life of the razor. The alcohol disinfects the blade and prevents rusting.

■ **Star Olive Oil.** After shaving your bikini line, apply Star Olive Oil to the area to prevent ingrown hairs.

■ **Vaseline Petroleum Jelly.** When you finish shaving, dip your safety razor blade in Vaseline Petroleum Jelly to prevent the blade from rusting, extending the life of your razor.

■ **WD-40.** To prolong the life of your safety razor blades, spray them with WD-40, a water-displacement formula that prevents the blades from rusting.

Immerse Yourself

■ Shave in the direction of the hair growth to avoid getting ingrown hairs.

■ The word *barbarian* means "unshaved." As the practice of shaving spread around the world, men in unshaved societies became known as barbarians, meaning "unbarbered."

■ Always shave during or after your take a shower or bath. The hot water softens the hairs, making them easier to shave.

■ Shaving does not cause the hair to grow back coarser and more quickly. When shaved hair begins to grow back, it initially appears

SKIPPY PEANUT BUTTER

In 1890, Dr. Ambrose W. Straub of St. Louis, Missouri, crushed peanuts into a paste for his geriatric patients with bad teeth. In 1903, Straub received the patent for a machine that grounded peanuts into butter, unveiling his invention at the 1904 World's Fair in St. Louis. By 1914, there were several dozen brands of peanut butter on the market.

In 1923, Joseph Rosefield perfected a process to prevent oil separation in peanut butter. Rosefield discovered that churning, rather than grinding peanuts, produced peanut butter with a much smoother consistency. After receiving the first patent for peanut butter that would stay fresh for up to a year, Rosefield joined forces with peanut butter manufacturer Swift & Company, known since 1928 as "Peter Pan." A dispute prompted Rosefield to leave the company, and in 1932, he started Rosefield Packing Company, in Alameda, California, to produce his own brand of peanut butter, which he named "Skippy." On February 1, 1932, Skippy Peanut Butter went on sale, and that same year, Rosefield added chopped peanuts to his product, introducing crunchy peanut butter.

thicker and coarser, but if allowed to grow, it regains its original appearance and texture.

■ A typical razor blade today is good for about ten shaves.

■ The average American man shaves twenty-four times per month, while the average American woman shaves eleven times per month.

■ Men use an average of thirty razor blades per year. Women use an average of ten blades per year.

■ The average man's beard has the same number of hairs as the average woman's legs and underarms combined.

■ A woman's underarm hair grows twice as fast as her leg hair.

Skin Problems

■ **Celestial Seasonings Green Tea.** To soothe reddened or irritated skin, steep three Celestial Seasonings Green Tea bags in a pot of boiled water and let cool. Saturate a washcloth in the tea and apply to the affected area for ten minutes, then rinse clean. Green tea is a natural anti-inflammatory.

■ **Fleischmann's Yeast** and **ReaLemon.** To tighten enlarged pores, mix the contents of one packet Fleischmann's yeast with enough ReaLemon lemon juice to make a thick paste. Apply the paste to your face, wait ten minutes, then rinse clean.

■ **McCormick Food Coloring** and **Lubriderm.** If your skin is red and chapped, you can cover up the appearance of redness by adding a drop or two of green food coloring to your moisturizer and then rubbing it into the reddened area.

■ **Scotch Tape.** Wrap some Scotch Tape around your finger, sticky-side out, and pat dry skin to exfoliate the flaky patches.

■ **Star Olive Oil, ReaLemon,** and **SueBee Honey.** Mix three tablespoons Star Olive Oil, four tablespoons ReaLemon lemon juice, and one tablespoon SueBee Honey is a sterilized jar and stir or shake well. Massage the mixture into dry elbows and ankles for two minutes, rinse clean, pat dry, and moisturize.

■ **Welch's 100% Purple Grape Juice.** Using a cotton ball, dab Welch's Grape Juice on your face to color your complexion. Wait one minute, then rinse.

ACNE

■ **Arm & Hammer Baking Soda.** Mix one teaspoon Arm & Hammer Baking Soda with enough water to make a paste. Put a small dab of the paste on any blemishes and let dry. The baking soda absorbs oils and dries the blemish.

■ **Bayer Aspirin.** Unless you're allergic to aspirin, grind six Bayer Aspirin into a fine powder using a mortar and pestle. Add enough water to make a thin paste and apply a dab of the paste on pimples. Salicylic acid, the main ingredient in aspirin, is also the primary ingredient in many commercial acne creams and skin cleansers.

■ **Colgate Toothpaste.** Apply a dab of Colgate Regular Flavor Toothpaste (not gel) on the pimples. The calcium carbonate in the toothpaste dries up pimples quickly and the glycerin soothes the skin. Just be sure to use the regular flavor—not the tartar control, which contains harsher chemicals.

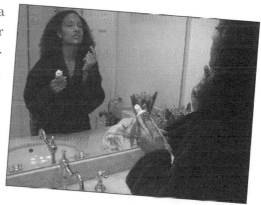

■ **Dannon Strawberry Yogurt.** Spread Dannon Strawberry Yogurt (mixed well) over your clean, dry face, wait five minutes, then rinse clean and pat dry. The salicylic acid in the strawberries, the same ingredient found in most commercial acne treatments, heals blemishes, and the lactic acid in the yogurt, smoothes your skin.

■ **Dannon Yogurt** and **Tidy Cats.** Mix one cup Dannon Plain Yogurt with one cup Tidy Cats Regular Clay to make a thick, muddy paste. Using a paint brush or spatula, spread the mud evenly over your face, gently massaging the mixture into your skin. Wait a half hour for the mud to dry. Rinse clean with warm water, followed by a quick rinse with cold water. Pat dry with a towel. The clay from the cat box filler detoxifies your skin by absorbing dirt and oil from the pores, while the yogurt soothes your skin.

■ **Dickinson's Witch Hazel.** Use a cotton ball dampened with Dickinson's Witch Hazel to clean oil from the skin. This astringent cleanses and tightening pores and also acts as an antiseptic.

■ **Elmer's Glue-All.** To remove blackheads, wash your face with soap and warm water, pat dry with a towel, and then coat your face with a thin layer of Elmer's Glue-All (avoiding your eyes). Let the glue dry, then gently peel it off, extracting blackheads with it. Elmer's Glue-All is water soluble, so should any stick to your eyebrows, you can wash it off with warm water.

■ **Epsom Salt.** To remove blackheads, mix one teaspoon Epsom Salt, three drops iodine, and one-half cup boiling water. Let the solution cool, dampen strips of cotton in it, and apply the strips to the clogged pores. Repeat three or four times, reheating the solution if necessary. Gently unclog your pores, then apply an alcohol-based astringent.

■ **Fleischmann's Yeast, ReaLemon,** and **Band-Aid Bandages.** Mix the contents of one packet Fleischmann's yeast with enough ReaLemon lemon juice to make a thick paste. Apply the paste over a rising pimple, cover with a Band-Aid Bandage, and leave on overnight. The yeast causes the pimple to emerge, and the astringent lemon juice disinfects it.

■ **Fruit of the Earth Aloe Vera Gel.** Apply a dab of Fruit of the Earth Aloe Vera Gel to reddened blemishes to tame the redness. The soothing gel made from Aloe Vera leaves promotes healing.

■ **Heinz White Vinegar.** To prevent pimples, use a cotton ball to cleanse your face with equal parts Heinz White Vinegar and water, which adjusts your skin to the proper pH level.

■ **Hydrogen Peroxide.** After cleansing your face, put a small amount of hydrogen peroxide on a cotton ball and wipe over your face, toning your pores with this mild astringent.

■ **Kingsford's Corn Starch** and **ReaLemon.** To dry up pimples and reduce redness, apply a paste made from one teaspoon Kingsford's Corn Starch and one teaspoon ReaLemon lemon juice, and let dry, then rinse. The cornstarch absorbs oil and brings pimples to a head, and the astringent lemon juice disinfects them.

■ **Knox Gelatin.** To eliminate blackheads, dissolve one tablespoon Knox Gelatin in two tablespoons milk over low heat. Let cool, then use a cotton ball to apply the mixture to your face, avoiding the eyes. Wait thirty minutes, then peel off the mask, exfoliating a thin layer of skin and removing blackheads with it.

■ **Lipton Tea Bags.** To bring a pimple to a head quickly, dampen a Lipton Tea bag with warm water and apply as a compress. The tannic acid absorbs the oils and dries the skin.

■ **Lipton Chamomile Tea Bags.** To clean pores and eliminate blackheads, fill a large bowl with boiling water and steep three Lipton Chamomile Tea Bags. Wearing a towel over your head to form a tent over the bowl, hold your face close to the steaming tea for ten minutes. When the tea cools, dampen a washcloth with the tea and cleanse your face, rubbing in circles. Rinse clean with cool water and moisturize.

■ **Listerine.** After washing your face with warm water and soap, use a cotton ball dampened with original flavor Listerine (not Cool

Mint, which contains sugar) to cleanse your pores, then dab it on blemishes. Wait ten minutes, then rinse your face with warm water to open the pores, followed by cool water to close the pores.

■ **Maalox.** Use a cotton ball to dab some Maalox on pimples. The antacid helps balance the pH of your skin and dry up excess oil.

■ **McCormick Ground Turmeric.** Mix one teaspoon McCormick Ground Turmeric with enough water to make a paste. Apply to blemishes and let set overnight.

■ **Minute Maid Orange Juice** and **SueBee Honey.** Mix one-half cup Minute Maid Orange Juice and one-half cup SueBee Honey. Apply to your face, avoiding your eyes. Wait five minutes, then rinse clean. The citric acid in the orange juice dries up excess oil, and the honey prevents bacteria from reproducing.

■ **Morton Salt.** Dissolve one teaspoon Morton Salt in one cup warm water. Dampen a cotton ball with the saline solution and hold it firmly against the blemish for a few minutes. The salt water reduces swelling and redness.

■ **Neosporin.** To clear up pimples, put a small dab of Neosporin on the blemish. The antibiotic kills bacteria and speeds healing.

■ **Ocean Spray Cranberry Juice Cocktail.** Soak gauze pads or a cotton handkerchief in Ocean Spray Cranberry Juice Cocktail and place it over your face, avoiding your eyes. Wait ten minutes, then rinse clean with warm water. Cranberry juice gently exfoliates dead skin and fights acne.

■ **Phillips' Milk of Magnesia.** Use Phillips' Milk of Magnesia as a facial mask to absorb oils from your face and dab it on pimples to reduce redness and speed healing. Let dry, then rinse clean.

■ **Preparation H.** Reduce the swelling and redness of pimples by applying a dab of Preparation H, a vasoconstrictor renowned for its ability to shrink inflammation.

■ **Quaker Oats.** Make a bowl of oatmeal according to the directions on the canister, let cool to the touch, and apply the warm oatmeal to your face (steering clear of the eyes). Cover with a washcloth dampened with warm water. Wait fifteen minutes, then wash clean. Repeat daily for one week, or whenever acne flares up. Oatmeal is a natural astringent that dries oils from the skin.

■ **Quaker Oats, Dannon Yogurt, ReaLemon,** and **Star Olive Oil.** Mix two tablespoons ground Quaker Oats, six tablespoons Dannon Plain Yogurt, two tablespoons ReaLemon lemon juice, and two teaspoons Star Olive Oil in a bowl. Apply the mixture to your face with your fingertips and massage gently over your face for five minutes. Rinse clean with warm water, followed by cold water, and pat dry with a towel. Repeat three times a day.

■ **ReaLemon.** Using a cotton ball, dab ReaLemon lemon juice over blackheads before going to bed. In the morning, wash off the juice with cool water. Repeat nightly until you notice sufficient progress in the condition of your skin. (Just be sure to stay out of the sun. The citric acid in lemon juice makes your skin more susceptible to sunburn.)

■ **Smirnoff Vodka** and **ReaLemon.** Mix one teaspoon Smirnoff Vodka and one teaspoon ReaLemon lemon juice and using a cotton ball, dab the mixture on pimples. The lemon juice is a natural antiseptic that disinfects the pores, and the alcohol in the vodka dries out the pimples.

■ **SueBee Honey** and **Band-Aid Bandages.** To bring an embedded pimple to a head, cover the blemish with a dab of SueBee

Honey and a Band-Aid Bandage. Honey inhibits bacteria, keeps the pimple sterile, and speeds healing, bringing the pimple to the surface overnight.

■ **SueBee Honey** and **Gerber Bananas.** Mix one teaspoon Sue-Bee Honey and one egg white, apply the mixture to your face, let dry, and then rinse clean. Apply the contents of one six-ounce jar Gerber Bananas to your face, wait ten minutes, then rinse clean.

■ **Vicks VapoRub.** A small dab of Vicks VapoRub applied to blemishes dries up the pimples.

■ **Visine.** Dampen a cotton ball with a few drops of Visine and touch it to the pimple or blemish for twenty seconds. Visine, a fast-acting vasoconstrictor, reduces the redness. (If you intend to use the eye drops in your eyes, do not let the tip of the bottle touch your skin.)

■ **Wonder Bread.** Soak a piece of Wonder Bread in milk and apply to the blemish for fifteen minutes. Rinse clean and pat dry.

FRECKLES AND SUNSPOTS

■ **Coppertone.** Avoid getting freckles and sunspots by wearing a sunscreen lotion such as Coppertone that has a sun protection factor (SPF) of at least 15 and that blocks both UVA and UVB rays. Be sure to reapply the sunscreen throughout the day. Freckles are caused by an accumulation of the skin pigment melanin, which responds unevenly to sunlight.

■ **Dannon Yogurt, ReaLemon, and Gold's Horseradish.** Mix one tablespoon Dannon Plain Yogurt, one teaspoon ReaLemon lemon juice, and one teaspoon Gold's Horseradish in a bowl. In a second bowl, mix one egg white and one teaspoon ReaLemon lemon juice and stir together over a saucepan of simmering water until the mixture thickens. Remove from heat, let cool, and then add to the yogurt mixture and stir well. Spread the mixture over freckled skin and let set for two hours. Rinse clean with warm water, pat dry with a towel, and moisturize the skin well.

■ **Gold's Horseradish, Heinz Apple Cider Vinegar,** and **Mr. Coffee Filters.** Place one tablespoon Gold's Horseradish in a bowl and use the spoon to spread out the horseradish evenly. Pour just enough Heinz Apple Cider Vinegar into the bowl to cover the horseradish. Let sit for ten days, then strain through a Mr. Coffee Filter. Dilute the liquid with an equal amount of water and use a cotton ball to apply to freckles and sun spots twice a day to minimize them (and in some cases, make them disappear completely). Store the remaining liquid in an airtight container.

■ **ReaLemon.** Apply ReaLemon lemon juice to the freckles or sunspots, wait fifteen minutes, then rinse clean. Lemon juice bleaches skin safely. (Using citric acid on your skin makes you more prone to sunburn, so be sure to use sunscreen afterward.)

WRINKLES

■ **Alberto VO5 Conditioning Hairdressing.** Before going to bed, rub a dab of Alberto VO5 Conditioning Hairdressing around your eyes to help prevent dry lines.

■ **Castor Oil.** To help prevent wrinkles around your eyes, rub castor oil around your eyes before going to bed at night.

■ **Carnation Nonfat Dry Milk** and **ReaLemon.** In a saucepan, mix three ounces Carnation Nonfat Dry Milk powder, one-cup water, and two teaspoons ReaLemon lemon juice. Bring to a boil, then let cool until warm to the touch. Use a pastry brush to paint the mixture over your face, neck, and chest. Let dry, then rinse with warm water. The lactic acid in the milk and the alpha-hydroxy acids in the lemon juice exfoliate dead skin, erasing wrinkles.

■ **Coppertone.** Wrinkling, discoloration, pronounced blood vessels, and cancerous lesions can be caused by prolonged exposure to the sun. To protect your skin from the sun, apply Coppertone sunscreen with a sun protection factor (SPF) of at least 15 at least thirty minutes before going outside in the sun.

■ **Crisco All-Vegetable Shortening.** Apply Crisco All-Vegetable Shortening as a salve on your face and hands every night before going to bed to moisturize the skin, keeping it soft, smooth, and healthy.

■ **Preparation H.** This cream not only shrinks hemorrhoids, but it also moisturizes skin, shrinks puffiness around your eyes, and reduces fine wrinkles around your eyes. Rub a small dab of Preparation H over wrinkles and puffy areas (without getting any in your eyes) to tighten skin and make fine lines vanish for several hours.

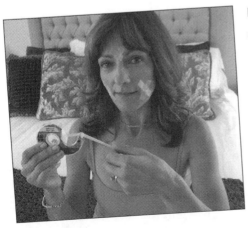

■ **Scotch Tape.** Frownies, small adhesive patches used to diminish wrinkles naturally, are applied to the face wherever you have frown or smile lines you wish to reduce. Left on while sleeping or relaxing and used over a period of two to four weeks, Frownies help retrain your muscles and smooth the frown and smile lines in your face. You can achieve the same effect by criss-crossing two small pieces of Scotch Tape between your eyebrows at night or over smile lines.

■ **Star Olive Oil** and **Heinz Apple Cider Vinegar.** To prevent wrinkles, mix two teaspoons Star Olive Oil and one teaspoon Heinz Apple Cider Vinegar. Rub the ointment into your face to keep the skin moisturized and supple.

Immerse Yourself

■ Stress, anxiety, fear, depression, or anger alter your hormones, which then clog pores, producing blemishes on the skin. Reduce stress by creating a relaxing atmosphere at home—with scented candles and tranquil music.

■ Drinking plenty of water flushes toxins from your system, rejuvenating skin and keeping it free from blemishes.

■ Poor dietary habits aggravate acne. Avoid processed foods containing additives and eat plenty of fresh fruits and vegetables.

■ Although excess sebum oil trapped in the passageways under the skin blocks the pores (causing pimples and blackheads to form), stripping away the excess sebum oil from the skin does not reduce acne. Instead, it causes the sebaceous glands to produce more sebum oil, creating the bacterial infection that causes pimples.

■ The best way to prevent acne is to gently wash dirt from the acid mantle of the skin.

■ As people age, hormone levels decrease, causing the sebaceous glands to produce less sebum to nourish the skin, increasing fine lines and wrinkles. Moisturizers help keep skin soft and hydrated, and facial scrubs exfoliate dead skin cells and stimulate cell renewal.

■ Vitamin C helps the body form collagen, the gluey fibers that hold skin taut. However, the skin does not necessarily absorb topical applications of Vitamin C deeply enough to affect collagen production. The best way to get Vitamin C into the body is by eating fresh fruits and vegetables. Vitamin C is also an antioxidant, and stable topical formulations, applied directly to the skin, protect it from UV damage caused by prolonged sun exposure.

■ Eating fruits and vegetables helps fight off free radicals, molecules that cause wrinkling, sagging, and age spots.

■ Exercise increases your circulation, creating new skin cells, and brings blood to the skin (putting color in your cheeks), and releasing perspiration, purging toxins from your body.

■ Avoid drinking alcohol. Alcohol dehydrates the body and dilates blood vessels, giving you a red nose.

■ Skin damaged by the sun produces more melanin, resulting in sunspots.

■ Even if you're wearing sunscreen, stay out of the sun when the sunlight is strongest and most direct—between 10 A.M. and 2 P.M.

■ UVA rays from the sun penetrate the dermis, cracking and shrinking the collagen and elastin, causing the epidermis to prematurely wrinkle and sag. UVB penetrate the epidermis and cause most skin cancers.

■ Wearing perfume when you're outside in the sun can result in spot burns wherever you've dabbed perfume on your skin.

■ Protection from sunscreen lasts only a few hours. Reapply the sunscreen as needed—especially after swimming or perspiring.

■ Apply sunscreen thirty minutes to an hour before going outside to give the sunscreen time to infuse your skin.

■ Contrary to popular belief, you can get a sunburn on a cloudy day. Ultraviolet rays from the sun penetrate clouds, no matter how overcast the sky may be.

■ To figure out how many hours of protection you can expect from a sunscreen, take the number of minutes it takes your skin to start burning without sunscreen, multiply by the sun protection factor (SPF) printed on the bottle of Coppertone, and divide the result by 60. For instance, if you usually burn in 30 minutes, an SPF 8 lotion should protect you for approximately 4 hours.

Stress Relief

■ **BenGay.** Massage a dab of BenGay into your temples to relieve tension throughout your body. The menthol in BenGay also provides an invigorating and uplifting dose of aromatherapy.

■ **Bubble Wrap.** If you're feeling tense and aggravated, grab a sheet of Bubble Wrap and use your thumb and index finger to pop the bubbles—one at a time. Popping Bubble Wrap is a harmless way to vent your anxiety and pent-up aggression, and it's amazingly therapeutic and fun to do.

■ **Crayola Crayons.** If you're under a lot of pressure or you're feeling nervous and edgy, grab a box of Crayola Crayons and draw a picture to express your feelings. Let your mind wander as your draw and use as many different colors as possible. You'll be amazed to discover how freely your subconscious fears, hostilities, and worries emerge in your drawing and your choice of colors. You'll purge many unhealthy feelings and gain startling insight into your emotions.

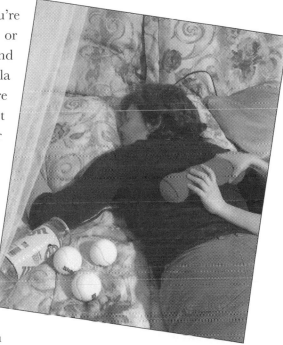

BENGAY

In 1898, French pharmacist Jules Bengué created a balm to soothe sore muscles and joints by combining menthol (for its heat-producing ability) and salicylate of methyl (an analgesic pain reliever) in a base of lanolin (for easy application). He named his product BenGay, after himself, and marketed the cream in Europe and America as a remedy for gout, rheumatoid arthritis, neuralgia, and stuffy sinuses from a head cold.

■ **Gold Medal Flour.** To make a stress balloon, stretch a balloon a few times, insert a funnel in the neck of the balloon, fill the balloon with Gold Medal Flour, and tie a knot. To relieve stress, simply squeeze the flour-filled balloon.

■ **Lipton Tea Bags.** Soothe tired eyes by immersing two Lipton Tea Bags in warm water, squeezing out the excess moisture, and placing them over your closed eyes for twenty minutes. The tannin in the tea reduces the puffiness and revitalizes tired eyes.

■ **McCormick Basil Leaves** and **Aunt Jemima Original Syrup.** If stress prevents you from falling asleep at night, bring three cups water to a boil, pour into a ceramic tea pot, and add one level teaspoon McCormick Basil Leaves. Cover and let steep for thirty minutes. Sweeten to taste with Aunt Jemima Original Syrup. Drink an hour before bedtime.

■ **Silly Putty.** Play with Silly Putty to calm your nerves and help tension disappear.

■ **Slinky.** Bouncing a Slinky between two hands has great therapeutic value in reducing emotional pressure and easing tension.

■ **SueBee Honey.** If stress keeps you awake at night, swallow one teaspoon SueBee Honey at bedtime. Honey acts as a sedative to the nervous system—usually within an hour. (Do not feed honey to infants under one year of age. Honey is a safe and wholesome food for older children and adults.)

■ **Wilson Tennis Balls.** Put several Wilson Tennis Balls inside a sock, tie a knot at the end, and have a friend roll this over your back. This technique is frequently used by labor coaches to massage the backs of women in labor.

Immerse Yourself

■ Stress, tension, and anxiety cause your adrenal glands to pump out stress hormones, such as adrenaline and cortisol, to deal with the situation. If your adrenal glands produce too many of these hormones, taxing your heart and weakening your immune system, you become susceptible to disease. These altered hormones can also clog pores and cause acne.

■ Before treating yourself to a home spa treatment, turn your home environment into a sanctuary to help clear your mind. Turn off the ringer on the telephone and turn off the volume on your answering machine so you can't be disturbed. Give yourself permission to enjoy time to yourself and forget about any deadlines for work or household chores that need to be done. Light scented candles, put out an assortment of plush towels, play soft music, and allow yourself to savor a home spa treatment. When you return to your work or chores, you'll feel restored and rejuvenated.

■ Trying to cope with stress by drinking coffee or alcohol can actually raise the levels of stress hormones in the blood, making you more tense and anxious.

■ Lighting scented candles, playing relaxing music, doing stretching exercises, and taking a soothing bath relieve stress.

Acknowledgments

At Fair Winds Press, I am grateful to my editor Ellen Phillips for her passion, enthusiasm, and excitement for this book. I am also deeply indebted to publisher Holly Schmidt, researcher and photo shoot producer Debbie Green, expert copy editor Jennifer Bright Reich, editorial assistant Ed Meagher, cover designer Laura McFadden, managing editor John Gettings, and proofreader Keith Powers .

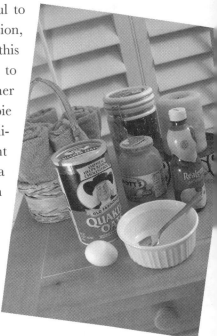

No amount of thanks can properly express my appreciation to talented models Laura Kotel, Maristella Dunn, Tiffany Barnes, makeup artist Victor Krone, and Debra Loggia for allowing us to photograph her home spa.

A very special thanks to my agent Jeremy Solomon, my manager Barb North, my Web site partner Michael Teitelbaum, and to the hundreds of people who constantly visit my Web site and send me their ingenious ideas.

Above all, all my love to Debbie, Ashley, and Julia.

The Fine Print

Sources

■ *All-New Hints from Heloise* by Heloise (New York: Perigee, 1989)

■ *Another Use For* by Vicki Lansky (Deephaven, Minnesota: Book Peddlers, 1991)

■ *Aroma Therapy: Essential Oils and How to Use Them* by Charla Devereux (London, England: Eddison Sadd, 2002)

■ *Ask Anne & Nan* by Anne Adams and Nancy Walker (Brattleboro, Vermont: Whetstone, 1989)

■ *The Bag Book* by Vicki Lansky (Deephaven, Minnesota: Book Peddlers, 2000)

■ *Baking Soda Bonanza* by Peter A. Ciullo (New York: HarperPerrenial, 1995)

■ *Bargain Beauty Secrets: Tips and Tricks for Looking Great and Feeling Fabulous* by Diane Irons (Naperville, Illinois: Sourcebooks, 2002)

■ *Beauty: The New Basics* by Rona Berg, Anja Kroencke, and Deborah Jaffe (New York: Workman, 2001)

■ *A Dash of Mustard* by Katy Holder and Jane Newdick (London: Chartwell Books, 1995)

■ *The Doctors Book of Home Remedies* by Editors of *Prevention* Magazine (Emmaus, Pennsylvania: Rodale Press, 1990)

■ *The Doctors Book of Home Remedies II* by Sid Kirchheimer and the Editors of *Prevention* Magazine (Emmaus, Pennsylvania: Rodale Press, 1993)

■ "Food for Thought—and Your Face" by Leslee Komaiko, *Los Angeles Times*, February 20, 2001, p. E1-3.

■ *Healing Home Spa: Soothe Your Symptoms, Ease Your Pain, and Age-Proof Your Body with Pleasure Remedies* by Valerie Gennari Cooksley

(New York: Prentice Hall, 2003)

■ *Heinerman's Encyclopedia of Healing Herbs & Spices* by John Heinerman (West Nyack, New York: Parker Publishing, 1996)

■ *The Herbal Home Spa: Naturally Refreshing Wraps, Rubs, Lotions, Masks, Oils, and Scrubs* by Greta Breedlove (North Adams, Massachusetts: Storey, 1998)

■ *Hints from Heloise* by Heloise (New York: Arbor House, 1980)

■ *Home Spa: Recipes and Techniques to Restore and Refresh* by Manine Rosa Golden (New York: Abbeville Press, 1997)

■ *Home Spa: Top-to-Toe Beauty Treatments for Total Well-Being* by Stephanie Donaldson (New York: Lorenz Books, 2002)

■ *The Home Spa: Creating a Personal Sanctuary* by Carol Endler Sterbenz (Kansas City: Andrews McMeel, 1999)

■ *Household Hints & Formulas* by Erik Bruun (New York: Black Dog and Leventhal, 1994)

■ *Household Hints for Upstairs, Downstairs, and All Around the House* by Carol Rees (New York: Henry Holt and Company, 1982)

■ *Household Hints & Handy Tips* by Reader's Digest (Pleasantville, New York: Reader's Digest Association, 1988)

■ *Jewish Literacy* by Rabbi Joseph Telushkin (New York: William Morrow, 1991)

■ *Kitchen Medicines* by Ben Charles Harris (Barre, Massachusetts: Barre, 1968)

■ *Make It Yourself: A Consumer's Guide to Cutting Household Costs* by Dolores Riccio and Joan Bingham (Radnor, Pennsylvania: Chilton, 1978)

■ *Mary Ellen's Best of Helpful Hints* by Mary Ellen Pinkham (New York: Warner/B. Lansky, 1979)

■ *Mary Ellen's Greatest Hints* by Mary Ellen Pinkham (New York: Fawcett Crest, 1990)

■ *Natural Home Spa* by Sian Rees (New York: Sterling, 1999)

■ *New Choices In Natural Healing: Over 1,800 of the Best Self-Help Remedies from the World of Alternative Medicine* by Bill Gottlieb (Emmaus, Pennsylvania: Rodale Books, 1997)

■ *911 Beauty Secrets: An Emergency Guide to Looking Great at Every Age, Size, and Budget* by Diane Irons (Naperville, Illinois: Sourcebooks, 1999)

■ *Panati's Extraordinary Origins of Everyday Things* by Charles Panati (New York: HarperCollins, 1987)

■ *Practical Problem Solver: Substitutes, Shortcuts, and Solutions for Making Life Easier* by Reader's Digest (Pleasantville, New York: Reader's Digest, 1991)

■ *Rodale's Book of Hints, Tips & Everyday Wisdom* by Carol Hupping, Cheryl Winters Tetreau, and Roger B. Yepsen, Jr. (Emmaus, Pennsylvania: Rodale Press, 1985)

■ *Spa: Pamper Body and Soul with Ideas from the World's Best Sources* by Karena Callen (New York: Rizzoli, 2001)

■ *Spa: Refreshing Rituals for Body and Soul* by Leslie Wolski (New York: Atria, 2003)

■ *The Spa Encyclopedia: A Guide to Treatments & Their Benefits for Health & Healing* by Hannelore R. Leavy and Reinhard R. Bergel, Ph.D. (Clifton Park, New York: Delmar Learning, 2003)

■ *The Spa Life at Home* by Margaret Pierpont and Diane Tegmeyer (Atlanta, Georgia: Longstreet Press, 1997)

■ *Spa Magic: Create a Spa at Home—with Healing, Rejuvenating, and Beautifying Recipes from Spas Around the World* by Mary Muryn (New York: Perigee, 2002)

■ *Vinegar: Over 400 Various, Versatile & Very Good Uses You've Probably Never Thought Of* by Vicki Lansky (Minnetonka, Minnesota: Book Peddlers, 2004)

■ *Weekend Home Spa: Four Creative Escapes—Cleansing, Energizing, Relaxing, and Pampering* by Linda Bird (Berkeley, California: Ulysses Press, 2001)

■ *The Woman's Day Help Book* by Geraldine Rhoads and Edna Paradis (New York: Viking, 1988)

■ *The World's Best-Kept Beauty Secrets* by Diane Irons (Naperville, Illinois: Sourcebooks, 1997)

■ *The World Book Encyclopedia* (Chicago: World Book, 1985)

Trademark Information

"Absorbine Jr." is a registered trademark of W.F. Young, Inc.

"Adolph's" is a registered trademark of Lipton, Inc.

"Afrin" is a registered trademark of Schering-Plough HealthCare Products, Inc.

"Ajax" is a registered trademark of Colgate-Palmolive.

"Albers" is a registered trademark of Nestlé Food Company.

"Alberto VO5" is a registered trademark of Alberto-Culver USA, Inc.

"Alka-Seltzer" is a registered trademark of Miles, Inc.

"Aqua Net" is a registered trademark of Faberge USA Inc.

"Arm & Hammer" is a registered trademark of Church & Dwight Co., Inc.

"Aunt Jemima" is a registered trademark of the Quaker Oats Company.

"Bacardi" is a registered trademark of Barcardi & Company Limited.

"Bag Balm" is a registered trademark of Dairy Association Co, Inc.

"Baker's" is a registered trademark of Kraft Foods, Inc.

"Balmex" is a registered trademark of Macsil Inc.

"Ban" is a registered trademark of Chattem, Inc.

"Band-Aid" is a registered trademark of Johnson & Johnson.

"Bayer" is a registered trademark of Bayer Corporation.

"BenGay" is a registered trademark of Pfizer Inc.

"Betty Crocker" and "Potato Buds" are registered trademarks of General Mills, Inc.

"Bigelow" and "Plantation Mint" are registered trademarks of R. C. Bigelow, Inc.

"Birds Eye" is a registered trademark of Birds Eye Foods.

"Blue Diamond" is a registered trademark of Blue Diamond Growers.

"Bounce" is a registered trademark of Procter & Gamble.

"Bounty" is a registered trademark of Procter & Gamble.

"Bubble Wrap" is a registered trademark of Sealed Air Corporation.

"Budweiser" is a registered trademark of Anheuser-Busch, Inc.

"C&H" is a registered trademark of C&H Sugar Company, Inc.

"Campbell" is a registered trademark of Campbell Soup Company.

"Canada Dry" is a registered trademark of Cadbury Beverages Inc.

"Carnation" is a registered trademark of Nestlé Food Company.

"Celestial Seasonings" is a registered trademark of the Hain Celestial Group, Inc.

"ChapStick" is a registered trademark of A. H. Robbins Company.

"Cheerios" is a registered trademark of General Mills, Inc.

"Cheez Whiz" is a registered trademark of Kraft Foods.

"Clairol" and "Herbal Essences" are registered trademarks of Clairol.

"Clean Shower" is a registered trademark of Church & Dwight Co., Inc.

"Clorox" is a registered trademark of The Clorox Company.

"Close-Up" is a registered trademark of Chesebrough-Ponds USA, Co.

"Coca-Cola" and "Coke" are registered trademarks of The Coca-Cola Company.

"Colgate" is a registered trademark of Colgate-Palmolive.

"Comet" is a registered trademark of Procter & Gamble.

"Conair" and "Pro Styler" are registered trademarks of Conair Corporation.

"Cool Whip" is a registered trademark of Kraft Foods.

"Coppertone" is a registered trademark of Schering-Plough HealthCare Products Inc.

"Cortaid" is a registered trademark of Pharmacia & Upjohn Company.

"Country Time" and "Country Time Lemonade" are registered trademarks of Dr Pepper/Seven Up, Inc.

"Crayola" is a registered trademark of Binney & Smith Inc.

"Crest" is a registered trademark of Procter & Gamble.

"Crisco" is a registered trademark of Procter & Gamble.

"Cutex" is a registered trademark of MedTech.

"Dannon" is a registered trademark of the Dannon Company.

"Dawn" is a registered trademark of Procter & Gamble.

"Dentyne" is a registered trademark of Warner-Lambert Co.

"Dial" is a registered trademark of The Dial Corp.

"Diamond" is a registered trademark of Diamond of California.

"Dickinson's" is a registered trademark of Dickinson Brands Inc.

"Dole" is a registered trademark of Dole Food Company, Inc.

"Downy" is a registered trademark of Procter & Gamble.

"Dr. Bronner's Peppermint Soap" is a registered trademark of All-One-God-Faith, Inc.

"Dynasty" is a registered trademark of JFC International, Inc.

"Easy Cheese" is a registered trademark of Nabisco.

"Easy-Off" is a registered trademark of Reckitt Benckiser, Inc.

"Efferdent" is a registered trademark of Warner-Lambert.

"Elmer's Glue-All" and Elmer the Bull are registered trademarks of Borden.

"Fantastik" is a registered trademark of S.C. Johnson & Sons, Inc.

"Febreze" is a registered trademark of Procter & Gamble.

"Fleischmann's" is a registered trademark of ConAgra Brands, Inc.

"Fleischmann's" is a registered trademark of ACH Foods, Inc

"Forster" is a registered trademark of Diamond Brands, Inc.

"French's" is a registered trademark of Reckitt Benckiser, Inc.

"Fruit of the Earth" is a registered trademark of Fruit of the Earth, Inc.

"Gatorade" is a registered trademark of The Gatorade Company.

"Gerber" is a registered trademark of Gerber Products Co.

"Gillette" and "Foamy" are registered trademarks of The Gillette Company.

"Glad" is a registered trademark of First Brands Corporation.

"Gold Medal" is a registered trademark of General Mills, Inc.

"Gold's" is a registered trademark of Gold's Pure Food Products Company, Inc.

"Grapeola" is a registered trademark of Kusha, Inc.

"Guinness" is a registered trademark of Diageo Guinness USA.

"Hain" is a registered trademark of Hain Pure Foods.

"Heinz" is a registered trademark of H.J. Heinz Company.

"Hennessy" is a registered trademark of Jas Hennessy & Co.

"Hershey's" is a registered trademark of Hershey Foods Corporation.

"Hodgson Mill" is a registered trademark of Hodgson Mill.

"Huggies" is a registered trademark of Kimberly-Clark Corporation.

"Hunt's" is a registered trademark of Hunt-Wesson, Inc.

"International Collection" is a registered trademark of Aarhus United UK Ltd.

"Ivory" is a registered trademark of Procter & Gamble.

"Jell-O" is a registered trademark of Kraft Foods.

"Jet-Puffed" is a registered trademark of First Brands International.

"Johnson's," "Johnson & Johnson," and "No Tears" are registered trademarks of Johnson & Johnson.

"Kingsford's" is a registered trademark of Bestfoods.

"Kleenex" is a registered trademark of Kimberly-Clark Corporation.

"Knox" is a registered trademark of NBTY, Inc.

"Knudsen" is a registered trademark of Kraft Foods.

"Kodak" is a registered trademark of Eastman Kodak Company.

"Kool-Aid" is a registered trademark of Kraft Foods.

"Kraft" is a registered trademark of Kraft Foods.

"Krazy" is a registered trademark of Borden, Inc.

"L'eggs" and "Sheer Energy" are registered trademarks of Sara Lee Corporation.

"Land O Lakes" is a registered trademark of Land O Lakes, Inc.

"Libby's" is a registered trademark of ConAgra Foods, Inc.

"Lipton," "The 'Brisk' Tea," and "Flo-Thru" are registered trademarks of the Thomas J. Lipton Company. "Listerine" is a registered trademark of Warner-Lambert.

"Loriva" and "nSpired Natural Foods" are registered trademarks of nSpired Natural Foods.

"Lubriderm" is a registered trademark of Warner-Lambert.

"Lysol" is a registered trademark of Reckitt Benckiser Inc.

"Maalox" is a registered trademark of Novartis Consumer Health, Inc.

"MasterCard" is a registered trademark of MasterCard International Inc.

"Maxwell House" and "Good to the Last Drop" are registered trademarks of Maxwell House Coffee Company.

"Maybelline" and "MoistureWhip" are registered trademarks of Maybelline.

"McCormick" is a registered trademark of McCormick & Company, Inc.

"Mennen" is a registered trademarks of The Mennen Co.

"Minute Maid" is a registered trademark of The Coca-Cola Company.

"Miracle Whip" is a registered trademark of Kraft Foods.

"Morton" is a registered trademark of Morton International, Inc.

"Mott's" is a registered trademark of Mott's USA.

"Mr. Coffee" is a registered trademark of Mr. Coffee, Inc.

"Mrs. Stewart's" is a registered trademark of Luther Ford & Company.

"Neosporin" is a registered trademark of Warner-Lambert.

"Nestea" is a registered trademark of Nestlé.

"Noxzema" is a registered trademark of Procter & Gamble.

"Ocean Spray" is a registered trademark of Ocean Spray Cranberries, Inc.

"Orajel" is a registered trademark of Del Laboratories, Inc.

"Oral-B" is a registered trademark of Oral-B Laboratories.

"Orville Redenbacher's" and "Gourmet" are registered trademarks of Hunt-
    Wesson, Inc.

"Palmolive" is a registered trademark of Colgate-Palmolive Company.

"Pam" is a registered trademark of American Home Foods.

"Pampers" is a registered trademark of Procter & Gamble.

"Parsons'" is a registered trademark of Church & Dwight Co., Inc.

"Pepto-Bismol" is a registered trademark of Procter & Gamble.

"Phillips'" is a registered trademark of Bayer Corporation.

"Playtex" and "Living" are registered trademarks of Playtex Products, Inc.

"Popsicle" is a registered trademark of Good Humor-Breyers Ice Cream.

"Post-it" is a registered trademark of 3M.

"Preparation H" is a registered trademark of Whitehall-Robbins.

"Purell" is a registered trademark of Gojo Industries, Inc.

"Q-Tips" is a registered trademark of Chesebrough-Pond's USA Co.

"Quaker Oats" is a registered trademark of the Quaker Oats Company.

"ReaLemon" is a registered trademark of Eagle Family Foods, Inc.

"ReaLime" is a registered trademark of Eagle Family Foods, Inc.

"Reddi-wip" is a registered trademark of ConAgra Brands, Inc.

"Reynolds," "Reynolds Wrap," and "Cut-Rite" are registered trademarks of
    Reynolds Metals.

"Right Guard" is a registered trademark of The Gillette Company.

"R.W. Knudsen" is a registered trademark of Knudsen & Sons, Inc.

"Saran Wrap" and "QuickCovers" are registered trademarks of S. C. Johnson &
    Son Inc. in the United States and Canada.

"Scotch-Brite," "Scotch" and "3M" are registered trademarks of 3M.

"Scrubbing Bubbles" is a registered trademark of S.C. Johnson & Son Inc.

"7 Up" is a registered trademark of Dr Pepper/Seven-Up, Inc.

"Sharpie" is a registered trademark of Sanford.

"Shout" is a registered trademark of S.C. Johnson & Sons, Inc.

"Silk" is a registered trademark of White Wave, Inc.

"Silly Putty" is a registered trademark of Binney & Smith Inc.

"Skin-So-Soft" is a registered trademark of Avon Products.

"Skippy" is a registered trademark of Unilever.

"Slinky" is a registered trademark of James Industries.

"Smirnoff" is a registered trademark of United Vintners & Distributors.

"S.O.S" is a registered trademark of The Clorox Company.

"Speed Stick" is a registered trademark of The Mennen Co.

"Spic and Span" is a registered trademark of Procter & Gamble.

"Sprite" is a registered trademark of The Coca-Cola Company.

"Star" is a registered trademark of Star Fine Foods.

"Static Guard" is a registered trademark of Alberto-Culver USA, Inc.

"Stayfree" is a registered trademark of McNeil-PPC, Inc.

"SueBee" is a registered trademark of Sioux Honey Association.

"Tabasco" is a registered trademark of McIlhenny Company.

"Tang" is a registered trademark of Kraft Foods.

"Thai Kitchen" is a registered trademark of Epicurean International, Inc.

"Tide" is a registered trademark of Procter & Gamble.

"Tidy Cats" is a registered trademark of the Ralston Purina Company.

"Tiger Balm" is a registered trademark of Haw Par Corporation Limited.

"Trojan" is a registered trademark of Carter-Wallace, Inc.

"20 Mule Team" and "Borax" are registered trademarks of United States Borax & Chemical Corporation.

"Uncle Ben's" and "Converted" are registered trademarks of Uncle Ben's, Inc.

"USA Today" is a registered trademark of Gannett News Service.

"Vaseline" is a registered trademark of the Chesebrough-Pond's USA.

"Vicks" and "VapoRub" are registered trademarks of Procter & Gamble.

"Visine" is a registered trademark of Pfizer, Inc.

"WD-40" is a registered trademark of the WD-40 Company.

"Welch's" is a registered trademark of Welch Foods Inc.

"Wesson" is a registered trademark of Hunt-Wesson, Inc.

"Wilson" is a registered trademark of Wilson Sporting Goods Co.

"Wonder" is a registered trademark of Interstate Brands Corporation.

"Woolite" is a registered trademark of Reckitt & Colman Inc.

"Ziploc" is a registered trademark of S. C. Johnson & Son Inc.

Index

for facials, 35
for hair styling, 94
Epsom salts
about, 57
for acne, 122
for baths, 7
for foot care, 45
in hair conditioning, 21
for hydrotherapy, 53
for nail care, 76
in rubs and scrubs, 104
as shampoo, 110
essential oils, in aromatherapy, 5

Fleischmann's Margarine
in hair conditioning, 25
for massage, 80
for moisturizing, 88
Fleischmann's yeast, for skin problems, 120, 122
flotation tank, 53
Forster Toothpicks, for nail care, 69–70
freckles and sunspots, 126–127
French's Mustard
for baths, 7
for facials, 35
for foot care, 45
for massage, 80–81
in mud packs and body wraps, 98
Fruit of the Earth Aloe Vera Gel
for acne, 122
in eye care, 29–30
for facials, 35
for foot care, 45
for hair styling, 94
for massage, 81
for moisturizing, 88
in mud packs and body wraps, 98
in rubs and scrubs, 106
for tooth care, 65

Gatorade
for hydrotherapy, 54
for lip care, 60
for massage, 81
for rehydration, 58
Gerber Bananas
for acne, 126
in eye care, 30
for facials, 36, 40
Gerber Carrots
for facials, 36
in rubs and scrubs, 102
Gerber Peaches, for facials, 36
Gerber Pears, in hair conditioning, 21
Gillette Foamy, for hair styling, 94
Glad Trash Bags, in mud wraps and body wraps,
97–98, 99, 101
Glycerin, for facials, 37
Gold Medal Flour
for facials, 36, 37, 11

in mud packs and body wraps, 100
as shampoo, 112–113
for stress relief, 132
Gold's Horse Radish
for freckles, 126–127
for massage, 81
Grapeola Grape Seed Oil
for massage, 81
for moisturizing, 88
Guinness Extra Stout, in hair conditioning, 21

Hain Safflower Oil
for baths, 7
in hair conditioning, 21
for massage, 82
for moisturizing, 88
Heinz Apple Cider Vinegar
for baths, 7
for cleansing and toning, 14
for facials, 41
for freckles, 127
in hair conditioning, 21, 22, 24
for mouth care, 63
in mud packs and body wraps, 98, 100
for nail care, 69
as shampoo, 110–111
for wrinkles, 129
Heinz White Vinegar
for acne, 123
for baths, 10
for cleansing and toning, 16
for foot care, 45
in hair conditioning, 19, 21–22
for nail care, 70–72, 75
as shampoo, 111
for shaving, 116
Hennessy Cognac, for facials, 37
Hershey's Cocoa, in mud packs and body wraps,
98
Hodgson Mill Wheat Germ, in rubs and scrubs,
104
Huggies Baby Wipes
for baths, 7
for hair care, 113
Hunt's Tomato Paste, for facials, 37
Hydrogen peroxide
for acne, 123
for cleansing and toning, 16
for mouth care, 63
for nail care, 72

ice packs, 55
International Collection Sweet Almond Oil
for bathing, 7
for facials, 42
in hair conditioning, 22
for lip care, 60
for massage, 80, 82
for moisturizing, 88
in mud packs and body wraps, 100

in rubs and scrubs, 104, 107
Ivory dishwashing liquid
for baths, 7–8

Jell-O
in eye care, 30
for foot care, 45, 46
for hair styling, 94
for ice packs, 55
for lip care, 60
for nail care, 72
Jet-Puffed Marshmallows, for nail care, 72
Johnson's Baby Oil
in aromatherapy, 2
for baths, 8, 9
for hair styling, 94
in hand care, 50, 51
for lip care, 61
for moisturizing, 89
for nail care, 72
in rubs and scrubs, 106
for shaving, 116
Johnson's Baby Powder
in hair removal, 27
in hand care, 50, 51
for massage, 82
as shampoo, 113
for shaving, 116
Johnson's Baby Shampoo, for facials, 33

Kingsford's Corn Starch
for acne, 123
for baths, 6
for facials, 35
for foot care, 45–46
in hair conditioning, 23
in hair removal, 26
for moisturizing, 89
in mud packs and body wraps, 98
for nail care, 72
as shampoo, 113
Kleenex Tissues, in cleansing and toning, 12
Knox Gelatin
for acne, 123
in hair conditioning, 21
in rubs and scrubs, 102
as shampoo, 111
Knudsen Sour Cream, for facials, 40
Kool-Aid, for lip care, 60
Kraft Mayo, in hair conditioning, 22
Krazy Glue
for nail care, 73, 74

Land O Lakes Butter
for massage, 82
for moisturizing, 89
for shaving, 116
L'eggs Sheer Energy Panty Hose
in aromatherapy, 2
for baths, 8, 9, 10

hair care and, 113
for hydrotherapy, 53–54
for ice packs, 55
in rubs and scrubs, 104–105, 107
Libby's Pumpkin
for facials, 37
in mud packs and body wraps, 99
in rubs and scrubs, 105
Lipton Chamomile tea
for acne, 123
for baths, 8
in eye care, 29
for facials, 36, 37
for hydrotherapy, 53–54
Lipton Tea Bags
for acne, 123
in eye care, 30
in hair conditioning, 22
in hair removal, 27
for lip care, 61
for mouth care, 62
for nail care, 73
for shaving, 116
for stress relief, 132
for tooth care, 65
Listerine
for acne, 123–124
for foot care, 46
for razor care, 116
as shampoo, 111
for tooth care, 65
Loriva Extra Sunflower Oil
for cleansing and toning, 13
for massage, 82
for moisturizing, 89
Lubriderm
for foot care, 45
for massage, 82–83
for nail care, 74

Maalox, for acne, 124
MasterCard
for mouth care, 63
for nail care, 74
Maxwell House Coffee
for baths, 9
for facials, 38
in mud packs and body wraps, 99
in rubs and scrubs, 105
Maybelline Clear Nail Polish, 73
Maybelline MoistureWhip Lipstick
for lip care, 61
tips for selecting, 66
McCormick Alum, for cleansing and toning, 16
McCormick Basil Leaves
in aromatherapy, 2
for stress relief, 132
McCormick Bay Leaves, in massage, 83
McCormick Cream of Tartar, for cleansing and
toning, 14

About the Author

Joey Green—author of *Polish Your Furniture with Panty Hose, Paint Your House with Powdered Milk, Wash Your Hair with Whipped Cream,* and *Clean Your Clothes with Cheez Whiz*—showed Barbara Walters how to prevent dehydration by putting a wet Pampers diaper on her head. He got Rosie O'Donnell to mousse her hair with Jell-O, gave Wayne Brady a facial with Pepto-Bismol, showed Dianne Sawyer how to condition hair with Cool Whip, and got Meredith Vieira to shave her legs with Cheez-Whiz. He has been seen polishing furniture with SPAM on *NBC Dateline*, cleaning a toilet with Coca-Cola in the *New York Times*, and washing his hair with Reddi-wip in *People*.

Green, a former contributing editor to *National Lampoon* and a former advertising copywriter at J. Walter Thompson, is the author of more than thirty books, including *Joey Green's Gardening Magic, Joey Green's Incredible Country Store, Joey Green's Amazing Kitchen Cures,* and *Joey Green's Magic Brands.* A native of Miami, Florida, and a graduate of Cornell University, he wrote television commercials for Burger King and Walt Disney World and won a Clio Award for a print ad he created for Eastman Kodak. He backpacked around the world for two years on his honeymoon and lives in Los Angeles with his wife, Debbie, and their two daughters, Ashley and Julia.

> **Visit Joey Green on the Internet at**
> **www.wackyuses.com**